International Perspectives on Primary Care Research

T0093692

International Perspectives on Primary Care Research

edited by

Felicity Goodyear-Smith
University of Auckland, New Zealand

Bob Mash
Stellenbosch University, Tygerberg, South Africa

On behalf of the **World Organization of Family Doctors** (WONCA)

With a Foreword by **Michael Kidd**, President of WONCA

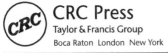

CRC Press
Taylor & Francis Group
Boca Raton London New York

CRC Press is an imprint of the
Taylor & Francis Group, an **informa** business

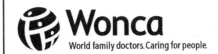

Wonca
World family doctors. Caring for people.

CRC Press
Taylor & Francis Group
6000 Broken Sound Parkway NW, Suite 300
Boca Raton, FL 33487-2742

© 2016 by Taylor & Francis Group, LLC
CRC Press is an imprint of Taylor & Francis Group, an Informa business

No claim to original U.S. Government works

Printed by CPI on sustainably sourced paper
Version Date: 20160115

International Standard Book Number-13: 978-1-78523-012-7 (Paperback)

This book contains information obtained from authentic and highly regarded sources. While all reasonable efforts have been made to publish reliable data and information, neither the author[s] nor the publisher can accept any legal responsibility or liability for any errors or omissions that may be made. The publishers wish to make clear that any views or opinions expressed in this book by individual editors, authors or contributors are personal to them and do not necessarily reflect the views/opinions of the publishers. The information or guidance contained in this book is intended for use by medical, scientific or health-care professionals and is provided strictly as a supplement to the medical or other professional's own judgement, their knowledge of the patient's medical history, relevant manufacturer's instructions and the appropriate best practice guidelines. Because of the rapid advances in medical science, any information or advice on dosages, procedures or diagnoses should be independently verified. The reader is strongly urged to consult the relevant national drug formulary and the drug companies' and device or material manufacturers' printed instructions, and their websites, before administering or utilizing any of the drugs, devices or materials mentioned in this book. This book does not indicate whether a particular treatment is appropriate or suitable for a particular individual. Ultimately it is the sole responsibility of the medical professional to make his or her own professional judgements, so as to advise and treat patients appropriately. The authors and publishers have also attempted to trace the copyright holders of all material reproduced in this publication and apologize to copyright holders if permission to publish in this form has not been obtained. If any copyright material has not been acknowledged please write and let us know so we may rectify in any future reprint.

Except as permitted under U.S. Copyright Law, no part of this book may be reprinted, reproduced, transmitted, or utilized in any form by any electronic, mechanical, or other means, now known or hereafter invented, including photocopying, microfilming, and recording, or in any information storage or retrieval system, without written permission from the publishers.

For permission to photocopy or use material electronically from this work, please access www.copyright.com (http://www.copyright.com/) or contact the Copyright Clearance Center, Inc. (CCC), 222 Rosewood Drive, Danvers, MA 01923, 978-750-8400. CCC is a not-for-profit organization that provides licenses and registration for a variety of users. For organizations that have been granted a photocopy license by the CCC, a separate system of payment has been arranged.

Trademark Notice: Product or corporate names may be trademarks or registered trademarks, and are used only for identification and explanation without intent to infringe.

Library of Congress Cataloging-in-Publication Data

Names: Goodyear-Smith, Felicity, editor. | Mash, Bob, editor.
Title: International perspectives to primary care research / editors:
Felicity Goodyear-Smith, Bob Mash.
Description: Boca Raton : Taylor & Francis/CRC Press, 2016. | Includes
bibliographical references and index. | Description based on print version
record and CIP data provided by publisher; resource not viewed.
Identifiers: LCCN 2015045101 (print) | LCCN 2015044027 (ebook) | ISBN
9781498767521 (e-book) | ISBN 9781785230127 (paperback : alk. paper)
Subjects: | MESH: Biomedical Research. | Primary Health Care--organization &
administration. | International Cooperation.
Classification: LCC R850 (print) | LCC R850 (ebook) | NLM W 84.61 | DDC
610.72/4--dc23
LC record available at http://lccn.loc.gov/2015045101

Visit the Taylor & Francis Web site at
http://www.taylorandfrancis.com

and the CRC Press Web site at
http://www.crcpress.com

Contents

Foreword

Research underpins the quality of clinical care we provide to our patients and to our communities. As health professionals, we are trained to practise medicine based on science and current knowledge. Our knowledge is based on the evidence provided by clinical research, the wisdom shared by our teachers and colleagues, and the insights that we gain from our daily work.

As clinicians, we are in the privileged position of being able to learn something new about human existence, health and disease every single day. I always think I have had a bad day in my clinical practice if I haven't learned something new from my patients or had a new research idea arising from something I have seen or heard. As a family doctor, my clinic is my laboratory. It is a source of new research ideas and observations. Research inspiration comes through the door of each of our clinics every single day.

Research is all about discovery. It can be great fun, and it can be very worthwhile. Every family doctor, every person working in primary care around the world, needs to be involved in primary care research. Our daily practice is based on research as we seek to translate new findings into our clinical care. As clinicians, we search the research literature for the evidence we need to provide the best care we can to our patients and our communities. We gain insights into our own practice and into the health issues facing our patient population through clinical audits. Many of us are involved in other peoples' research through completion of surveys or involvement in studies, and some of us conduct our own research, seeking to improve medical knowledge and lead the exploration of the boundaries of clinical medicine. Our involvement in research allows us to adapt to the changes that inevitably take place as medical practice evolves throughout our careers.

This new publication is a welcome addition to our library of great World Organization of Family Doctors publications. I thank the members of our World Organization of Family Doctors Research Working Party, led by editors Professor Felicity Goodyear-Smith from New Zealand and Professor Bob Mash from South Africa, for tackling this important challenge and producing a great new resource for international primary care. I thank the contributing authors from around the world for sharing their insights and their expertise. I am sure this will be a valuable resource for all primary care researchers; for policymakers and academics and journalists interested in the importance of primary care research; and for health science and medical students, research higher degree candidates and experienced researchers interested in joining us as new researchers in primary care.

Professor Michael Kidd, AM MBBS, MD, DCCH, FRACGP
President, World Organization of Family Doctors

and

Matthew Flinders Distinguished Professor and Executive Dean
of the Faculty of Medicine, Nursing and Health Sciences,
Flinders University, Adelaide, Australia

Editors

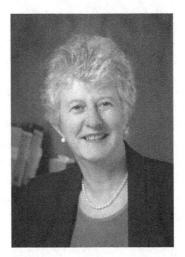

Felicity Goodyear-Smith is a general practitioner and academic head of the Department of General Practice and Primary Health Care, The University of Auckland, Auckland, New Zealand. She has over 200 papers in peer-reviewed journals, as well as a number of other publications, including three books and several book chapters. Felicity is passionate about the importance of research underpinning clinical practice in primary care, and supports the nurturing of primary care research globally. She was founding editor of the *Journal of Primary Health Care*, a peer-reviewed research journal designed to meet the information needs of New Zealand general practitioners, practice nurses and community pharmacists plus other primary healthcare practitioners. Started in 2009, the journal was MEDLINE listed after 12 months and has an impact factor of 0.76. She chairs the International Committee of the North American Primary Care Research Group and, in 2016, will take over the chair of the World Organization of Family Doctors Working Party on Research. In her spare time, Felicity likes to travel and enjoys hiking, swimming and kayaking.

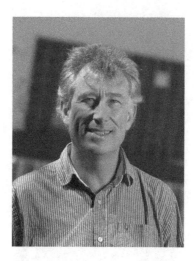

Bob Mash graduated from The University of Edinburgh and trained as a general practitioner in Scotland before emigrating to South Africa in 1991. He worked in the townships outside Cape Town with community health workers, providing community-based primary care in the final days of the apartheid era. Following the onset of democracy, he worked for 10 years in the public sector, providing primary care in Khayelitsha. During this period, he worked with Stellenbosch University to create the first learning opportunities in family medicine and primary care for undergraduate medical students. Subsequently, he also developed a new online master's degree programme for the training of family physicians.

He obtained his PhD on mental disorders in primary care in 2002 and has now published over 130 articles in peer-reviewed scientific journals. He is currently the head of Family Medicine and Primary Care at Stellenbosch University and responsible for research activities and training at both master's and doctoral levels. He is the editor-in-chief of the *African Journal of Primary Health Care & Family Medicine* and is a rated researcher with the National Research Foundation. He is a founding member of the Chronic Diseases Initiative for Africa (a network of researchers) and an active leader within the Primary Care and Family Medicine Education (Primafamed) Network, a group of departments of family medicine in sub-Saharan Africa. He is also a member of the World Organization of Family Doctors Working Party on Research.

Contributors

Faisal Abdullatif Alnasir, FPC, FRCGP, MICGP, FFPH, PhD
Professor
Department of Family and Community
  Medicine
Arabian Gulf University
Manama, Bahrain

Mehmet Akman, MD, MPH
Associate Professor
Department of Family Medicine
School of Medicine
Marmara University
Istanbul, Turkey

Magda Almeida, MD, MPH, FCFP
Professor
Department of Public Health
Faculty of Medicine
Federal University of Ceará
Fortaleza, Brazil

José Ramirez Aranda, MD, PhD
Professor
Department of Family Practice
Pedro de Alba S/N
Ciudad Universitaria
San Nicolás de los Garza
Nuevo León, Mexico

Tabinda Ashfaq, MBBS, FCPS
Assistant Professor
Department of Family Medicine
Aga Kahn University
Karachi, Pakistan

Olayinka Ayankogbe, MBBS
Senior Lecturer
Community Health and Primary Care
College of Medicine
University of Lagos
Lagos, Nigeria

Gillian Bartlett, PhD
Associate Professor
Research and Graduate Program Director
Department of Family Medicine
McGill University
Montreal, Canada

Sandro Rodrigues Batista, MSc
Assistant Professor
Department of Internal Medicine
Federal University of Goiás
Goiás, Brazil

Andrew Bazemore, MD
Director
Robert Graham Center Policy Studies in
  Family Medicine and Primary Care
Washington, DC, USA

John Beasley, MD
Professor of Family Medicine
Department of Family Medicine and
  Community Health
University of Wisconsin
Madison, Wisconsin, USA

Patrick Chege, MBChB, MMed
Senior Lecturer and Head
Department of Family Medicine
College of Health Sciences
Moi University
Eldoret, Kenya

Akye Essuman, MBChB, FWACP
Head of Family Medicine
University of Ghana
Accra, Ghana

Terry Findlay, MBus, B Soc Stud
Associate Professor
Australian Primary Health Care Research
  Institute
Australian National University
Canberra, Australia

Robert Fryatt, MBBS, MD, MPH, MRCP,
FFPHM
Public Health and Health Systems Specialist
London School of Hygiene and Tropical
  Medicine
London, UK

Felicity Goodyear-Smith, MBChB, MD,
FRNZCGP
General Practitioner and Academic Head
Department of General Practice and Primary
  Health Care
University of Auckland
Auckland, New Zealand

Larry Green, MD
Professor and Epperson Zorn Chair for
  Innovation in Family Medicine and Primary
  Care
University of Colorado
Denver, Colorado, USA

Gustavo Gusso, MD, TEMFC (SBMFC),
MClSci, PhD
Assistant Professor of General Practice
Universidade de São Paulo
São Paulo, Brazil

Jeannie Haggerty, PhD
Associate Professor and McGill Chair in
  Family and Community Medicine Research
Department of Family Medicine
McGill University
Montreal, Canada

Richard Hobbs, MA, FRCGP, FRCP, FESC,
FMedSci, FRCP
Professor and Head of Primary Care
Nuffield Department of Primary Care Health
  Sciences
University of Oxford, UK

Amanda Howe, MA, Med, MD, FRCGP,
FAcadMED
Professor of Primary Care
Norwich Medical School
University of East Anglia
Norwich, UK

Per Kallestrup, MD, PhD
Associate Professor
Department of Public Health
Aarhus University
Aarhus, Denmark

Khaled Karkabi, MD, MMH
Professor and Chair of the Department of
  Family Medicine
Faculty of Medicine
Technion – Israel Institute of Technology
Haifa, Israel

Tony Kendrick, MD, FRCGP, FRCPsych
(Hon)
Professor of Primary Care
Department of Primary Care and Population
  Sciences
University of Southampton
Southampton, UK

Michael Kidd, AM, MBBS, MD, DCCH,
FRACGP
President
World Organization of Family Doctors
and
Matthew Flinders Distinguished Professor
and
Executive Dean
Faculty of Medicine Nursing and Health
  Sciences
Flinders University
Adelaide, Australia

Raman Kumar, MBBS, DNB
President
Academy of Family Physicians of India
New Delhi, India

Christos Lionis, MD, PhD, FRCGP (Hons)
Professor of General Practice and Primary
  Care
Clinic of Social and Family Medicine
School of Medicine
University of Crete
Crete, Greece

Leslie London, MBChB, MMed, BSc (Hons),
FCPHM, MD
Professor
Division of Public Health Medicine
School of Public Health and Family Medicine
University of Cape Town
Cape Town, South Africa

Jan De Maeseneer, MD, PhD
Professor
Department of Family Medicine and Primary
  Health Care
Ghent University
Ghent, Belgium

Dee Mangin, MBChB, DPH, FRNZCGP
Associate Professor
Department of Family Medicine
McMaster University
Hamilton, Ontario, Canada

David Mant, OBE, MA, MBChB, FRCGP,
FRCP, FMedSci
Emeritus Professor of General Practice
University of Oxford
Oxford, UK

Bob Mash, MBChB, DRCOG, DCH, FRCGP
(UK), FCFP (SA), PhD
Head
Family Medicine and Primary Care
Stellenbosch University
Tygerberg, South Africa

Kevin McCarthy
Policy/International Aid-Cooperation Officer
European Commission
EuropeAid
Unit for Education, Health, Research and
  Culture, Health Sector
Brussels, Belgium

Ellen McIntyre, OAM
Professor
Discipline of General Practice
and
Director
Primary Health Care Research and
  Information Service
Flinders University
Adelaide, Australia

Sergio Minué, MD
Professor
Coordinator World Health Organization
  Collaborating Center on Integrated Health
  Services Based on Primary Health Care
Andalusian School of Public Health
Granada, Spain

Gboyega Ogunbanjo, MBBS, MFamMed,
FCFP
Head
Department of Family Medicine and Primary
  Health Care
University of Limpopo
Pretoria, South Africa

Wim Peersman, PhD
Professor
Department of Family Medicine and Primary
  Health Care
Ghent University
Ghent, Belgium

Elena Petelos, BSc (Hons), MPH, PhD
Clinic of Social and Family Medicine
School of Medicine
University of Crete
Crete, Greece

Luisa Pettigrew, MBChB, MRCGP, MSc
NIHR In-Practice Fellow
Faculty of Public Health and Policy
Department of Health Services Research and
  Policy
London School of Hygiene and Tropical
  Medicine
London, UK

William Phillips, MD, MPH
Theodore J Phillips Endowed Professor in
  Family Medicine
University of Washington
Seattle, Washington, USA

Jacqueline Ponzo, MD, MSC
Adjunct Professor
Department of Family and Community
  Medicine
Faculty of Medicine
University of the Republic
Uruguay

Joanne Reeve, BClinSci, MBChB, MPH,
PhD, FRCGP
Chair
Society for Academic Primary Care
and
Associate Clinical Professor in General
  Practice
University of Warwick
Coventry, UK

Rebecca Roper, MS, MPH
Initiative Lead Fellow
Agency for Healthcare Research and Quality
Practice-Based Research Network
and
National Center for Excellence in Primary
Care Research
Center for Evidence and Practice
Improvement
Washington, DC, USA

Sherina Mohd Sidik, MBBS, MMED, PhD
Professor
Family Medicine
Universiti Putra Malaysia
Kuala Lumpur, Malaysia

Clare Taylor, MB ChB, FRCGP
Academic Clinical Fellow
Nuffield Department of Primary Care Health
Sciences
University of Oxford
Oxford, UK

Thiago Trindade
Professor
Federal University of Rio Grande do Norte
Natal, Brazil

Mehmet Ungan, MD
Professor
Department of Family Medicine
Ankara University School of Medicine
Ankara, Turkey

Peter Vedsted, MD, PhD
Director and Professor
Department of Public Health and Department
of Clinical Medicine
Aarhus University
Aarhus, Denmark

Jim Warren, PhD
Professor of Health Informatics
The University of Auckland
Auckland, New Zealand

Chris van Weel, MD, PhD, FRCGP, FRACGP
Professor of Primary Health Care Research
Australian National University
Canberra, Australia
and
Emeritus Professor of Family Medicine /
General Practice
Radboud University Nijmegen
Nijmegen, Netherlands

**Carl de Wet, MBChB DRCOG FRCGP
FRACGP MMed**
General Practitioner and Senior Clinical
Lecturer
Logan Hyperdome Doctors
Loganholme, Australia
and
Griffith University
Gold Coast, Australia

Emma Whitehead, PGDp, MSc, BS (Hons)
Consultant to Australian Primary Health Care
Research Institute
Australian National University
Canberra, Australia

**William Wong, MD, MPH, FRACGP,
FRCGP**
Clinical Associate Professor and Chief of
Research
Department of Family Medicine and Primary
Care
University of Hong Kong
Hong Kong, China

Nick Zwar, MBBS, FRACGP, MPH, PhD
Professor
School of Public Health and Community
Medicine
University of New South Wales
Sydney, Australia

SECTION I

What is primary care research?

Introduction

Felicity Goodyear-Smith

In this section of our book on primary care research, I give a brief history of the development of research in the primary care setting as a discipline in its own right. John Beasley then presents a typology of primary care research, based on the initial work of Barbara Starfield. This broad scope of primary care enquiry, incorporating basic, clinical, health services, health systems and educational research, becomes the framework for later sections of the book.

Bob Mash describes the wide-ranging categories of professionals and academics who conduct primary care research, the types of methods used and how research capacity can be developed. Amanda Howe focuses on patient and public involvement in the research process, how this may be effective and the benefits it may confer. Finally, Jim Warren explains how the data from electronic primary care health records can be harnessed to answer a wide range of questions, using a variety of study designs, and possibly linking to other large datasets, in ways not previously possible with paper-based records.

CHAPTER 1

The history of primary care research

....

Felicity Goodyear-Smith

Compared with other medical disciplines, academic general practice has a very short history. The earliest use of the term 'general practitioner' appears to have been in 1809,[1] but it was soon in common use. In 1828, Professor Thomson of the Westminster Medical Society argued against medical specialisation when he wrote 'The general practitioner [should] be looked upon as at the head of the profession.'[2] However, most British medical practitioners were members of the Royal Colleges of Physicians or Surgeons or the Society of Apothecaries. Throughout the nineteenth until the mid-twentieth century, physicians and surgeons specialised and held hospital appointments, from which community-based doctors were largely excluded.[3] Despite several attempts, a college of general practitioners was not founded in Britain until 1952. The *College of General Practitioners' Research Newsletter*, in 1953, was the first publication of general practice research. It developed into the *Journal of the College of General Practitioners* and is now the *British Journal of General Practice*. It took another decade for the first chair in general practice to be established, which was in Edinburgh, Scotland in 1963. The first English chair in general practice was not founded until 1972 in Manchester.

It must be noted that different countries use different terminology. The term 'general practice' is generally synonymous with family medicine, and likewise 'general practitioner' with 'family doctor' or 'family physician'. The general scope is the holistic approach of caring for individuals and their families in the community, treating patients of both genders of all ages with every disease entity. An exception is in the USA, where the term 'family medicine' replaced 'general practice' in the 1970s, and 'general practitioner' now refers to a hospital-based general physician practising internal medicine.[4]

While the terms 'primary care' and 'primary healthcare' are often used interchangeably, 'primary care' applies to general practice–type services delivered to patients and their families, whereas 'primary healthcare' has a broader meaning, including service delivery, inter-sectorial collaboration to address the social determinants of health and community participation.[5] Primary care is not just medical care, as it is delivered by doctors, nurses, clinical officers, community health workers, community pharmacists and a number of other front-line and allied health professionals.[6]

This book uses the term 'primary care research' to refer to the body of knowledge generated in primary care or by primary care providers that intends to contribute to the improvement of people's health and well-being from this context. Primary care, of course, is situated within the broader understanding of primary healthcare, and research inevitably speaks to this broader approach to improving people's health.

In 1972, the World Organization of Family Doctors (WONCA) was founded by member organisations in 18 countries. WONCA's mission is 'to improve the quality of life of the peoples of the world through defining and promoting its values, including respect for universal human rights and including gender equity, and by fostering high standards of care in general practice/family medicine'. WONCA now has 118 member organizations in 131 countries.[7]

In 1978, the World Health Organization issued a declaration at Alma-Ata underlining the international importance of primary care. It stated that

> primary health care is essential health care based on practical, scientifically sound and socially acceptable methods and technology made universally accessible to individuals and families in the community through their full participation and at a cost that the community and country can afford to maintain at every stage of their development in the spirit of self-reliance and self-determination. It forms an integral part both of the country's health system, of which it is the central function and main focus, and of the overall social and economic development of the community. It is the first level of contact of individuals, the family and community with the national health system bringing health care as close as possible to where people live and work.[8]

The document also underlines the importance of primary care research: 'Primary health care ... is based on the application of the relevant results of social, biomedical and health services research and public health experience'.

Since the 1970s, there has been continuing growth in general practice / family medicine as an academic discipline. By 2000, there were 27 departments of general practice in UK medical schools. Initially, general practice academics found that teaching undergraduate and vocational training programmes, as well as maintaining heavy clinical workloads, took priority over research activities.[9] Furthermore, some general practitioners were appointed to senior academic posts without research degrees or significant contribution to peer-reviewed literature.[10] However, in university settings, transmission of knowledge should not be divorced from generation of knowledge. There was a rapid growth in the research culture, with the understanding that it informs both clinical practice and teaching, and that creation of new knowledge is a mark of an academic discipline. Departments developed doctoral programmes and became actively engaged in research.

This has been reflected in the growing body of research literature. There have been an increasing number of general practice / family medicine / primary care journals

TABLE 1.1 Primary care / General practice / Family medicine journals publishing original research

Journal	Founded	Language
College of General Practitioners' Research Newsletter (UK)	1953	English
Journal of the College of General Practice	1960	
Journal of the Royal College of General Practice	1967	
British Journal of General Practice	1990	
Canadian Family Physician	1954	English and French
Australian Family Physician	1972	English
New Zealand Family Physician	1974	English
Journal of Primary Health Care (New Zealand)	2009	
Hong Kong Practitioner	1978	English
South African Family Practice Journal	1980	English
Scandinavian Journal of Primary Health Care (Nordic countries)	1983	English
Family Practice (International)	1984	English
Revista Portuguesa de Medicina Geral e Familiar (Portugal)	1984	Portuguese
Malaysian Family Physician	1989	English
Utposten (Norway)	1995	Norwegian
Australian Journal of Primary Health	1995	English
Atención Primaria (Spain)	1996	Spanish
Türkiye Aile Hekimliği Dergisi (Turkey)	1997	Turkish
Journal of the American Board of Family Medicine	1998	English
Primary Health Care Research & Development (UK)	2000	English
Asia Pacific Family Medicine	2001	English
Chinese Journal of General Practitioners	2002	English and Chinese
Annals of Family Medicine (USA)	2003	English
Archivos de Medicina General y Familiar (Argentina)	2004	Spanish
Revista Médico de Familia (Venezuela)	2004	Spanish
Revista Brasileira de Medicina de Família e Comunidade (Brazil)	2004	Portuguese
Actualizatión en Medicina de Familia (Spain)	2005	Spanish
African Journal of Primary Health Care & Family Medicine	2009	English
Eurasian Journal of Family Medicine (Turkey)	2012	English and Turkish
Journal of Family Medicine and Primary Care (India)	2012	English
Chinese General Practice	2013	English and Chinese
Revista Mexicana de Medicina Familiar (Mexico)	2014	Spanish

published since the 1980s, with developing regions and countries starting their own, often in their own language, over the past decade (see Table 1.1). These publish a variable mix of original research plus continuing educational material for their clinical readers. Many were included in *Index Medicus* and are now included in MEDLINE. The primary consideration in selecting journals for indexing is the scientific merit of a journal's content. The validity, importance, originality and contribution to the coverage of the field of the overall contents are key factors considered by the National Library of Medicine's (NLM) selection panel in recommending a journal for indexing.[11]

In 2009, Professor Chris van Weel, past president of WONCA, facilitated the NLM to introduce the new subject heading 'Primary Health Care' (including family medicine) in *Index Medicus*, and journals that focus on general practice, family medicine and primary healthcare were reallocated to this subject.[11] It should be noted, of course, that primary care research is also published in general medical journals and a wide range of other discipline and condition-specific publications.

CHAPTER 2

The nature of primary care research

....

John Beasley, Andrew Bazemore and Bob Mash

Although research in primary care is often seen as being mainly clinical research, there are many opportunities, as well as a great need, to do research with a much broader scope to improve the health of individuals and populations in all countries.[12] A framework, originally articulated by Starfield[13] and added to by Mold and Green,[14] is useful to understand the potential broad scope of primary care research. This scope includes (with minor modifications from the original papers):

1. Basic research that focuses on the methods used to conduct research in primary care (e.g. What are the ways primary care research networks can be organised?[15]).
2. Clinical research that focuses on the diagnosis and treatment of clinical problems (e.g. Does long term treatment with azithromycin improve outcomes in asthmatics?[16]).
3. Health services research that explores factors that impact the way we deliver care and the organisation of clinical operations. This area is especially critical given the implementation of health information technology (e.g. What are the tasks performed by physicians in primary care encounters?[17]).
4. Health systems research explores the macro-scale economic and political factors that affect primary care.[18]
5. Educational research that has a focus on education for students and practitioners for primary care and the health workforce for primary care (e.g. What is the best training site for medical students for primary care careers?).[19]

The typology of primary care research just presented can be further expanded by considering whether the context of the research is the community served by the primary care team or the patients seen at the primary care facility. This contextual model (Table 2.1) expands the possibilities for primary care research. Community-oriented primary care acts as a bridge to the more traditional public health research that may be concerned with epidemiology and population health.

Bodies such as the USA's Institute of Medicine continue to emphasise the importance

TABLE 2.1 Context and primary care research typology

	Community oriented	**Facility oriented**
Basic	Research into the development of tools or methods for use in the household or community	Research into the development of tools or methods for use in the facility
Clinical research	Community burden of disease research using household data	Primary care morbidity research using patient records
	Investigating the prevention of disease in the community	Investigating the management of disease in the facility
Health services research	Research into the characteristics of community-based services such as coverage, health promotion and disease prevention	Research into the characteristics of facility-based services such as access, continuity, integration and comprehensiveness
Health systems research	Policy research in support of inter-sectorial action for upstream causes of disease	Policy research in support of better governance and financing of primary care services
Educational research	Research into the training of community health workers and primary healthcare teams	Research into the training of primary healthcare providers such as nurses or doctors

of context in defining 'primary care' as 'the provision of integrated, accessible health care services by clinicians, who are accountable for addressing a large majority of personal health care needs, developing a sustained partnership with patients, and practicing in the context of family and community'.[20] Moreover, just as primary care is needed globally, *Now More than Ever,*[21] to improve individual and population health, its research enterprise must also reflect increasing awareness of the importance of 'upstream', or social determinants critical to achieving those aims.

Some of this research will benefit greatly from collaborations with other disciplines, and, in fact, it is essential to draw on the expertise and resources that exist in other areas, while bringing our own expertise in primary care and ensuring that the questions asked and the methods used are appropriate to address important issues. While some of these collaborations will be with other medical disciplines, other collaborations are emerging that are particularly useful because the systems through which we deliver care change rapidly. As one example, collaborations with industrial and systems engineering are proving useful.[22]

Having this taxonomy, and the potential to partner with other disciplines, in mind helps to avoid a too-narrow focus on clinical research and will help enable a robust and diverse primary care research enterprise that will improve the health of persons in all nations. This taxonomy of primary care research has been used as our understanding of the field in writing and editing this book.

CHAPTER 3

Who conducts primary care research?

. . . .

Bob Mash

Primary care providers should play a much stronger role in shaping and conducting research in and about their own practice. Primary care providers, who are usually a mix of doctors, nurses and mid-level doctors, are often too busy handling the clinical workload to engage significantly with the research necessary to strengthen and improve primary care. In many countries, academic departments of family medicine and primary care have established a cadre of primary care providers who can champion relevant research. In low- and middle-income countries (LMICs), however, academic primary care providers may be overwhelmed with the responsibilities of teaching and lack more advanced research skills. Not all the disciplines involved in primary care have developed academic expertise, and this is especially true of mid-level workers and, to a lesser extent, primary care nurses. Building research capacity is therefore key to future success.

One of the most successful strategies for engaging large numbers of primary care providers is the formation of primary care research networks. Networks can allow grassroots practitioners to contribute to research throughout the country without the need to conceptualise and design the actual study, while, for the principal investigator, the network allows him or her to have a broad sampling strategy and large sample size. Examples of such networks are given in Section IV of this book.

Although primary care providers should be at the heart of primary care research, there are a large number of other disciplines that also contribute to the research agenda. During 2014, the following disciplines all published work in the *African Journal of Primary Health Care & Family Medicine*: family medicine, nursing, midwifery, nutrition and dietetics, pharmacy, psychology, optometry, speech and language, sociology, internal medicine, obstetrics and psychiatry. Similarly, the *Journal of Primary Health Care* included research from the disciplines of family medicine, public health, community pharmacy, primary care nursing, midwifery, clinical epidemiology, social and community health, sociology, psychology, health service delivery and health systems, health informatics and health economics. The range of clinical disciplines involved in primary care and the collaborative nature of general practice lend themselves to a similar collaborative approach to primary care research.

When the focus of primary care research moves away from clinical issues to health services, health systems and the social determinants of health, the range of potential researchers expands once again to include, for example, public health researchers, economists and informatics experts.

Transdisciplinary research that embraces researchers from outside the health sciences is also becoming important in tackling the complexity involved in the social determinants of health.

What types of research methods are used in primary care research?

This section outlines the range of research methods typically used in primary care research, although it does not attempt to teach the details of these methods. The different methods are discussed under three broad paradigms, which offer different epistemological approaches to the generation of new knowledge. The essential characteristics of these paradigms are shown in Table 3.1.[23] In reality researchers often combine methods derived from these different paradigms to fully answer their research question.

Scientific medicine has traditionally embraced the empirical-analytical research paradigm, and the evidence-based medicine movement has emphasised a hierarchy

TABLE 3.1 Epistemology of different research paradigms

Paradigm	Empirical-analytical	Interpretative-hermeneutic	Emancipatory-critical
Relationship of researcher to 'reality'	Testing and measuring	Exploring and interpreting	Changing and transforming
View of the researched person	Object to be measured	Subject to be understood	Participant in the process
View of truth	Correspondence to the facts	Coherence within the data	Consensus of each person's learning
Research process	Predominantly quantitative measurements	Predominantly qualitative measurements	Participatory using both quantitative and qualitative techniques
Research question	Fixed hypothesis	Open ended	Open ended
	Set by the researcher	Set by the researcher	Negotiated with group and can evolve
Implementation of results	Recommendations made for action by other people	Insights offered for use by other people	Findings implemented as part of the research
	Generalisable	Transferable	Transferable

of such research methods, with the synthesis of evidence from randomised controlled trials in systematic reviews at the pinnacle. Below this would come quasi-experimental studies, observational studies (such as cross-sectional, case-control and cohort studies) and, finally, case series or case reports. These research methods are all relevant to primary care research, although much of the evidence generated by clinical trials has been derived from hospital settings and study populations who are not typical of primary care. Primary care providers have criticised the evidence base, therefore, for not being entirely relevant to the type of clinical decisions, complexity and morbidity profile of primary care. There is a need for clinical questions derived from primary care practice to be addressed by well-designed trials conducted in primary care.

Another critique of the current evidence base is that trials are often conducted in ideal conditions and with highly selected patient groups (often excluding patients with co-morbidity or pregnancy and those who are adolescents or children). There is a need to not just test the efficacy of new therapies in such ideal situations but to evaluate their effectiveness in real-world primary care. The concept of such pragmatic clinical trials has gained ground as a way of evaluating interventions in normal health service conditions.[24]

Apart from developing and testing new approaches to clinical problems, there is also the need to take to scale and utilise in primary care practice what we already know. In fact, it has been argued that if we were to actually implement what we already know works, this would be a more effective use of our time. The gap between what we know works from previous research studies and actual clinical practice is huge, especially in LMICs in which primary care systems are weak. One way of trying to bridge this gap is the development and implementation of evidence-based guidelines. How to effectively implement new evidence in primary care practice has led to the growth of implementation science and translational research.

Quality improvement cycles are a common method used to engage practitioners with the latest evidence in an approach of action learning that encourages them to reflect on how to improve their practice, make the suggested changes and then evaluate the effect in continuous cycles. Quality improvement cycles may be embedded into the organisational practice of the health services, but, in many contexts, the lessons learned and the innovation created through this activity are worth sharing and have been published as original research.[25] Primary care research with a focus on quality improvement and improving patient safety is discussed in more detail in Chapter 8, by Carl de Wet, in Section II.

The biopsychosocial approach required of a generalist working in primary care and the need for person-centred care as a core feature of medical generalism[26] has also led primary care researchers to embrace other research methods. For example, questions arise in clinical practice regarding how patients experience care, how they make sense of illness, how they make decisions about seeking help or taking medication and what their preferences are in terms of treatment. These important questions cannot be explored adequately with methods derived from the empirical-analytical paradigm; instead, researchers have engaged methods derived from the interpretative-hermeneutic research paradigm. Such methods are qualitative and typically include participant observation, non-participant observation as well as qualitative interviewing via individual or group interviews.[27,28]

The desire to engage with communities and to work collaboratively in order to improve one's clinical practice and to solve problems in the real world has also led many researchers to explore the emancipatory-critical research paradigm. Action research has several traditions that are relevant to primary care.[29] The oldest of these is perhaps that of empowering participatory action research that has attempted to engage with communities and in a health context to enable them to understand their social determinants of health more deeply and to take action to address them. Empowering communities to understand and solve their own health problems is a powerful process; for instance, a rural community in South Africa addressed the problem of young men dying from complications of traditional circumcision.[30] Professional action research has a different focus and is usually conducted by a group of health professionals who wish to improve their own clinical practice. A good example of this approach is the cooperative inquiry group, which focuses on solving a specific question derived from clinical practice.[31] The principles of this approach have been described in the 'CRASP' model as:[32]

- **C**ritical collaborative inquiry by.
- **R**eflective practitioners being.
- **A**ccountable and making the results of their inquiry public.
- **S**elf-evaluating their practice and engaged in.
- **P**articipative problem-solving and continuing professional development.

The group simultaneously experiments with changing its practice while also observing what happens and learning both individually and collectively. A cyclical process enables both action and research to progress over time. Examples of action research are given in Chapter 4 by Amanda Howe.

In traditional clinical trials, different contexts are generally controlled or adjusted for, with the aim of working with homogenised populations (excluding outliers and non-typical settings) to reduce 'noise'. Recently, there has been a rise in implementation research to more accurately reflect 'real-life' community settings. This approach embraces heterogeneity and focuses on the integration of complex systems and the development of a framework to enable the scaling up of a programme, tailored to the specific needs of different settings and populations.[33] Rather than using logic models with linear links between inputs and outputs, implementation research employs the theory of change, allowing for diversity and the interaction and adaption of an intervention with its specific context. Its use of mixed methods may address 'intention to reach', rather than 'intention to treat', for equitable health impacts.[34] Building on the participatory research model, implementation research may develop democratic partnerships between researchers and community stakeholders. The aim is to involve end-users at the onset in framing questions, study design and delivery, and subsequent uptake of findings.[35] It seeks to empower participants to modify an intervention to suit their own context. Stakeholders may include patients and healthcare providers, as well as managers and policymakers and other key players. The co-creation approach places the end-user at its core and seeks to establish long-term collaborations between end-users and the researchers.[35,36]

How to develop research capacity

The number of established researchers in the field of primary care worldwide is relatively small. In LMICs especially, there is a need to develop capacity. In most LMICs, there are very few researchers with doctorates in family medicine or related disciplines. ESSENCE on Health Research has recently published seven principles for good practice in research-capacity strengthening in LMICs.[37] These are discussed following, with specific suggestions made by primary care researchers in the African context.[38]

'Network, collaborate, communicate and share experiences'

Building capacity in primary care research requires the development of national, regional and global networks to share expertise and best practice. The WONCA Working Party on Research has responsibility at a global level to foster such networking and collaboration. Regional networks such as the Primary Care and Family Medicine Education (Primafamed) Network in Africa can also enable people to share methodological and scientific expertise, find collaborators with similar interests or research questions, find supervisors or mentors, set strategic priorities and directions, as well as reach consensus on key issues to communicate to funders or government. One should not forget the need to include community members and front-line primary care providers in setting a research agenda. Partnerships with local policymakers and managers of the district health system can help to ensure the relevance of research questions and future buy-in of the health services to the results.

'Understand the local context and accurately evaluate existing research capacity'

An evaluation may be necessary to understand the research expertise in the local context and what capacity or capability is present or lacking. 'Capability' refers to the skills and competencies of the novice or emerging researchers and the training that may be needed to develop them as established researchers with the full methodological repertoire. 'Capacity' refers to the health services context as well as political, policy and economic climate, which may enable or hinder this emerging capability. This might include, for example, the emphasis placed on primary healthcare and universal coverage in government policy and the funds that are made available for research. Each academic department should have a clear strategy for its research priorities as well as research capacity building.

'Ensure local ownership and active support'

Research capacity building may require external expertise, but this should not undermine the need for local ownership of the process and direction. Local stakeholders, including communities, practitioners, academics, policymakers and researchers, should collaboratively identify the research gaps and needs to be addressed. In many countries, there is a need to advocate for support of primary care research and to motivate for funding of research that strengthens health services and systems and which is not just focused on specific diseases or biomedical questions. WONCA is in support of the 15 by 2015 campaign that challenges funders to commit 15% of their funding to the strengthening of health systems and services by 2015.[39]

'Build-in monitoring, evaluation and learning from the start'

If an intervention is planned to build research capacity the evaluation of that intervention should be planned from the start. Monitoring may include the number of people trained, for example, obtaining master's or doctoral degrees, or the number of publications in peer-reviewed scientific journals. However, the dominance of assessing research outputs based on the impact factor of journals may need to be balanced with the more meaningful evaluation of actual societal impact. Societal impact may be measured by the influence of research on policy or communities; for instance, presentation of the research to a lay audience, inclusion in policy, or inclusion in training curricula or guidelines.

'Establish robust research governance and support structures and promote effective leadership'

Primary care researchers should be supported by adequate local governance and support structures that assist with identifying potential funders, grant management and ethical review. The process of ethical review and permission to perform research should be made as efficient as possible. Emerging researchers should be developed not just for their scientific competence but also for their leadership ability. A variety of training opportunities should be offered for undergraduates and postgraduates at both master's and doctoral levels. Training should address the range of methods relevant to primary care as well as skills in scientific writing. Opportunities for presentation and incentives for publication should be available for both novice and established researchers. Requiring master's students to produce their research in the form of an original research article rather than a traditional thesis can increase the visibility of research and chance of publication.

'Embed strong support, supervision and mentorship structures'

Novice and emerging researchers need to be both supervised and mentored. Supervision may be from a more experienced researcher with expertise in the methodology, research topic or scientific writing. Mentorship is a more personal activity that helps the researcher to grow and develop. Both supervision and mentorship require an ability to give timely and useful feedback and effective coaching, in addition to sharing scientific expertise, and these interpersonal skills cannot necessarily be assumed to be automatically present with seniority. In LMICs, supervision and mentoring may need to happen at a distance, even from other countries. Co-supervision with a local more inexperienced supervisor and a distant more experienced supervisor can be a useful strategy to develop both the supervisor and the student.

'Think long-term, be flexible and plan for continuity'

Research capacity–building initiatives may require a long-term commitment and continuity over many years to create a lasting difference. Strategies should address both individual capability as well as the contextual issues that enable capacity and should rely on diversified funding sources within an overarching strategic framework.

CHAPTER 4

Effective patient involvement in research: why, who and how?

....

Amanda Howe

INTRODUCTION

The purpose of most medical research is to find ways to improve people's health or test the outcomes of new clinical interventions and treatments. In primary care research, we particularly focus on the individual patient, rather than a specific disease, body system or technique. We rely on patients to say 'yes' when asked to help us with research, whether the project involves letting us access their clinical data, take a simple blood test, have a one-to-one interview or follow them up over a period. In this age in which the rights of the individual are paramount, ethical practice in research is essential and full information sharing and informed consent are a requirement of clinical research, who better to help us ensure that our research is designed with the needs of patients in mind than patients themselves?

Many countries and research funders now require patient and public input into research – both on ethics committees and specific research projects. But the literature on how to do this effectively is only just emerging, and many researchers and patients would say this 'sounds like a good idea, but what does it mean in practice?' This chapter summarises findings from some recent research and gives some principles for practice that you may want to consider when drawing up systems and protocols for your own research setting.

PATIENT AND PUBLIC INVOLVEMENT: DEFINITIONS AND DIMENSIONS

Various words can be used to describe people who contribute to research but are neither academics nor clinical staff – 'patients', 'public', 'laypersons' and 'community members' all appear in the English-language literature. It is important to note that such people are not the same as the 'research participants' – that is, the people who are the subjects of the research study and have agreed to participate in the research. Patient and public involvement (PPI) leads are there to advise and guide the researchers, not as the subjects of the research.

There are different types of involvement and stages of patient input. PPI leads can:

- Comment on ideas and priorities for research.
- Comment on specific proposals and how they may work best for patients.
- Read and provide feedback on information sheets and consent forms to make sure they really explain the research and what is involved in a way that other members of the public will understand.
- Discuss findings and their implications as they emerge from the project.
- Help to spread the findings in a way that is valuable to, and understandable by, the public.
- Act as co-researchers, if suitably trained, doing interviews and collecting data – again, this may be very helpful to get access to some communities who would not willingly confide in professional staff.
- Be a whole community or sector of the population that act as co-researchers. This last form, community-based participatory research (CBPR), is a 'collaborative approach to research that equitably involves all partners in the research process and recognizes the unique strengths that each brings. CBPR begins with a research topic of importance to the community, has the aim of combining knowledge with action and achieving social change to improve health outcomes and eliminate health disparities'.[40]

In PPI, the key issue is the role that is played rather than the background of the person. For example, a retired nurse could be on a research project to give views about what patients might expect – the important thing is that she or he is there to speak for patients and their families, not as a researcher with a specific research interest. One area of particular controversy is whether members of the public in such a setting are 'representative'. There may be projects in which this is truly the case – for example, when a community chooses specific people to link with a research team who is working in their setting – but one or two people on a research project can rarely reflect the specific cultural perspectives of the many ages, races and patient groups who primary care research might involve. So it is important that these people first see their role as thinking of patient perspectives beyond their own experience and come prepared to give a 'voice for patients'. It is also important that researchers get different types of public involvement – being on an ethics committee and commenting on many different projects requires a different skill set than does engaging with specific groups to enhance the research.

For example, a patient lead might question whether any patients will be involved who cannot read or write, and advocate for ensuring that the researchers provide pictorial explanations of the project or translations into other languages and formats, if needed. He or she might also test the expectations of the researchers as to whether the research will make too many demands of the patients involved – 'Are you really expecting the patients to come to the clinic six more times just for the research assessments? Can't you arrange to do them while they are attending their routine appointments?' But if there are specific groups on which more in-depth understanding is needed, some way needs to be found for those groups to feed in. An example might be a project researching why young people have run away from home: here, the 'patient rep' will be more use if they are from that community or have some links into it, and can help to advise how the researchers might access the young people – and what will be needed to make it 'safe' for them to talk to the researchers. So there are many choices to be made about who makes the PPI input and how this is best done.

WHY HAVE PATIENT INVOLVEMENT?

There are two main reasons: a moral one – that research is being done for patients and on patients, so they should have some voice in this and appropriate protections; and a practical one – that it will make the research better and more effective. Of course, the way in which this expertise is drawn into the research setting also matters. There is evidence that this can work well through different types of involvement: (1) long-term (as in members who are recruited to advise on multiple projects over a prolonged period), (2) periodic – at specific stages of a project, and (3) outreach based – to engage communities and patients to get specific advice and insights. All of these can work well, but there are some conditions that may make this more or less effective.

WHAT HELPS (OR HINDERS)?

In discussion with laypeople who have become active in PPI or CBPR, it is clear that this can be a very enabling experience – interesting, rewarding and enhancing skills and understanding for both academic researchers and the community or lay members. It can also be challenging – dynamics of power, knowledge, resource use and priorities can be played out, as with any other human interaction. Clarity of purpose, clear goals and managing expectations are key both to work with individuals and communities. Recent research suggests the following:[41]

- The researchers themselves need to be committed to having a patient voice on the team and to listening to her or his views: they also need to explain the project in a way that PPI leads can understand.
- Both the researchers and the patient / community leads will benefit from training about what their roles and relationships need to involve; the members of the public will need to have some understanding of the research project and process to make sense of what their comments need to focus on.
- Having a named person as the main contact between the researchers and the patient reps helps with communication and coordination.

- Being clear about the roles of each person is important, but with flexibility if these need to be developed or altered over time.
- Resources will need to be put aside by organisations or research projects for public involvement costs – training, travel, other agreed costs (e.g. carers' backfill) and time.
- Relationships really matter! This will not be news to family doctors, but it is a key finding that full public involvement in research is facilitated by ensuring that the member of the public or community is treated as a valued part of the research team and its efforts.

Relationships must first be established face to face before more remote but functional forms of communication, such as email, can be utilised effectively. A mechanistic or utilitarian approach by researchers is not appreciated by those trying to advocate for other patients.

CONCLUSION

Just as the days of the patriarchal authority of the doctor are (or should be) past, so is the autocracy of the scientific expert. We need to do research for the benefit of our patients, taking their views and needs into account, and have people working with us as researchers who can hold the patient's 'gaze' as their main purpose and responsibility. Public involvement in research can add value to the planning, process and outputs of primary care research, providing it is done in a way that is practical, personally committed and properly resourced. It can also be a force for social change. This is a learning process for all of us – and, as we know, sometimes our patients are our greatest teachers!

CHAPTER 5

Primary care research in the digital age: unleashing the power of electronic patient records

Jim Warren

GROWTH OF THE PRIMARY CARE ELECTRONIC MEDICAL RECORD

Use of computers in patient consultations is now a routine part of primary care in many settings globally. Terminology around such systems varies, including 'electronic health record' (EHR) and 'electronic medical record' (EMR), the former suggesting aspects of health and wellness, not just medicine. A recent survey, however, considered a basic EHR to be a system that can: record patient history and demographics, maintain patient problem lists, record clinical notes, record medication and allergy lists, view laboratory results and imaging reports and do prescription ordering.[42] As these are rather 'medical' functions, we will refer to a computerised system providing these patient record capabilities as an 'EMR system' and the data managed by such a system as 'the EMR'.

The proportion of US physicians reporting they use EMRs has risen from 46% in 2009 to 69% in 2012[43] – a rise that corresponds to massive federal incentives for 'meaningful use' of such systems.[44] Many parts of the world saw such growth earlier and already stood at 95%-plus rates of uptake in 2009, including Australia, the Netherlands, New Zealand, Norway and the UK.[45] For example, in Australia, a national programme incentivised electronic prescribing and connectivity in general practice in the late 1990s, leading to a 90% uptake of EMR systems by 2005.[45] EMR systems are also being taken up in the developing world; in sub-Saharan Africa as a case in point, use is dominated by open-source software – to avoid prohibitive procurement costs – and often focuses on HIV treatment programmes.[46]

Uptake and sustained use of EMR systems in primary care creates large collections of local data at each practice. Although subject to legislative and ethical challenges, there is potential for integration of records across practices and for primary care systems to interoperate with other health sector systems and, increasingly, with applications used by patients themselves. This chapter unpacks the concept of the primary care EMR and its research potential.

PROVENANCE AND SEMANTICS IN THE ELECTRONIC MEDICAL RECORD

A primary care EMR provides a rich picture of individual patient cases with a range of applications. Actual collection of data from an EMR system is often simple from an IT perspective: the systems typically provide reporting functions, including 'advanced' functions to extract data using the International Organization for Standardization Structured Query Language, creating output compatible with spreadsheet or statistical packages. Primary care EMR data elements are easily misinterpreted, however, especially when analysts are not themselves directly familiar with use of the EMR system in daily practice. Researchers must pay careful attention to the 'provenance' (i.e. source) and 'semantics' (exact meaning in context) for EMR data elements.

Table 5.1 consolidates issues in terms of positive predictive value (PPV), and, broadly, what it means for a datum to be present for a case; and negative predictive value, and what it means for a datum to be absent. Electronic prescribing data illustrate many key points. If a prescription record is present in the EMR, we can be confident a primary care provider prescribed the indicated medication (good PPV), and the information should be sufficiently precise and accurate for the pharmacist to dispense. Discrepancies can still arise (e.g. a telephone discussion between doctor and pharmacist can result in changes not updated to the EMR) but are rare and often minor. To the extent that the date of prescription is recent, relative to the duration of the prescription, we can take this as a current medication. Data flags may be present to indicate stopped medications or other changes, but reliability is limited by whether users are rigorous in completing such fields. On the other hand, the absence of a prescription is limited as an indicator that a patient is not on that medication – they may receive prescriptions from other providers in the community or through secondary care. In some settings, an e-pharmacy network exists providing data on prescriptions by other providers and for dispensing (e.g. as through the Danish Medicines Agency for general practitioners in Denmark[47]), but this is not the general case.

Similar reasoning about provenance and semantics must be applied for research use of other EMR components, with further problems emerging in terms of format and selection bias. For instance, coding schemes are well-established for primary care users to select classifications of problems – such as using the World Health Organization's *International Classification of Disease* or the *International Classification of Primary Care* (developed by WONCA and allowing classification of reason for encounter and management, as well as problem).[48,49] A physician may find encoding a problem in 'free-text' notes sufficient for purposes of delivering care but that extraction of the un-coded problem from the notes requires application of natural language processing (NLP) algorithms. These algorithms are becoming increasingly effective in interpreting free-text notes to extract information such as the temporal history of events and indications for medications;[50] such NLP tools are not yet, however, part of the typical health researcher's toolkit. Laboratory tests illustrate selection bias. The test result itself is likely to be reliable, although care has to be taken with differences in test names and units between testing services. Test orders are not, however, uniformly distributed across the patient population; there are biases: (1) towards patients whose condition is

TABLE 5.1 Types of primary care electronic medical record (EMR) data elements and their interpretation

Data elements	Positive predictive value (PPV) and validity	Negative predictive value and completeness
Patient history, allergies and demographics	Good PPV for general categories of events; but filtered by patient	Largely limited by what patient recalls and chooses to share
Patient problem lists	Good PPV but possibly limited by primary care context and coding system	Largely unreliable – mostly discretionary to code problems (except 'notifiable' conditions) and not all problems are necessarily known
Clinical notes/ observations	Potentially good PPV but, unless coded, require hand or machine extraction of specific data*	Limited by completeness of recording, ability to extract facts from descriptions and what is presented at consult
Current medications / prescriptions	Prescriptions very reliable – if the EMR shows a prescription, the patient is very likely to have received that prescription. Current medications also reliable, as based on prescribing if date of last prescription considered	Limited – does not include prescriptions made by other providers; for long-term medication started in the EMR, cessation or gaps have moderate reliability for detecting non-adherence[52]
Laboratory results and imaging reports	Very reliable – if a result is recorded then a test was done and the result is probably valid; imaging record often codes type of imaging but reports are limited similarly to clinical notes	Limited – tests may have been done, and many may not have been sent to primary care or have been recorded in structured format in the EMR
Letters – incoming (e.g. hospital discharge) and outgoing (e.g. referral)	Generally only unstructured content except for date and source/destination	Limited to the extent that discharges might not be reported to the practice, or referrals could be made by other providers

*Potential for recording bias (recording abnormal but not normal findings) limiting inference of patterns; also possible rounding.

more critical being tested more frequently than those achieving 'normal' values, and (2) against timely testing of patients less engaged with the healthcare system (e.g. certain ethnicities participating in screening to lower levels than others[51]). The assumption that missing values are randomly distributed is not defensible.

PUTTING THE DATA TO WORK

Table 5.2 summarises applications in which the primary care EMR can support research. The EMR can support any initiative, from practical rollout of a procedural change to a formal randomised controlled trial (RCT). First, the EMR can be queried, creating a list of eligible participants to be contacted for recruitment. Moreover, some EMRs support user-programmable prompts, allowing notification for recruitment to appear on the physician's desktop when an eligible patient presents.[53] Secondly, the EMR can be periodically queried during a study to support monitoring for adverse effects. Thirdly, the EMR can be queried at the end of a study to provide outcome measures (e.g. change in a physiological measure from baseline versus treatment period). However, this use is limited by biases noted in the previous subsection, 'Provenance and semantics in the EMR'. When it is not practical to organise an RCT, propensity score methods allow observational studies to mimic characteristics of an RCT.[54] For example, if an EMR spans multiple clinics, a subset of which undertook an intervention, comparison cases can be selected from non-intervention sites matched in terms of key characteristics like age and condition severity.

In the context of condition-specific registries, the EMR can be queried to create a registry used for further action. Queries can also be used to identify gaps in recorded data. In conducting such queries, care must be taken to distinguish 'null' values (absence of data) from negative value (e.g. explicit observation that a patient is a non-smoker). Particularly if followed up by expert manual review of the EMR contents including free-text notes, such an analysis constitutes an audit and may serve as a starting point for a drive for more complete information or as evaluation of an intervention expected to have led to more complete information.

The EMR can support descriptive and exploratory studies. Detection of unwarranted regional variation in healthcare delivery was pioneered by Jack Wennberg.[55] EMRs from even a small set of primary care practices can be used to assess quality and variation in practice. The primary care EMR can also feed public health monitoring.[56] A further potential application of primary care EMRs is post-market pharmacovigilance (e.g. detecting association of medication uptake with increased rate of hospitalisation). This role is best served by 'data-mining' algorithms that search broadly for emergent patterns, since the analyst cannot fully specify the unanticipated adverse event. Such functions have been demonstrated on administrative data sets[57] – their use on primary care EMRs would be made more powerful with data linkage.

There are obvious research benefits to the linkage of primary care EMRs to other data sets – for example, to capture hospitalisation and mortality events not systematically stored in primary care. But barriers to data linkage arise from privacy concerns.

TABLE 5.2 Applications of the primary care electronic medical record to research

Application	Description
Study recruitment	Identification of eligible participants (to form a register, or on a rolling basis as patients present)
Study monitoring	Monitoring for elevated rates of negative outcomes
Study evaluation	Assessing levels of the dependent variable in treatment and control groups; propensity score methods to reduce confounding
Registry formulation and improvement	Identification of a set of cases eligible for an intervention, or identification of cases in need of further data collection; assessment of registry completeness
Monitoring variation, epidemiology and public health	Forming descriptive models of management or outcome levels, changes (including pharmacovigilance and sudden changes characteristic of outbreaks) or differences (e.g. by demographics, geography or provider)

In the US, context standards for acceptable data management are defined by the Health Insurance Portability and Accountability Act (HIPAA) Privacy Rule, which requires de-identification of data shared in research networks.[58] The HIPAA allows re-identification risk to be mitigated by various methods, including perturbation of data values. El Emam[59] reviews de-identification methods, including the introduction of random noise into the counts of patients satisfying a query, as well as maintenance of audit trails with limits on related queries that could be used to estimate the mean of perturbed data. Wider inclusion of primary care EMRs in such privacy-preserving linkage has great potential for enhancing their research value.

DIRECTIONS IN PRIMARY CARE DATA

The present-day primary care EMR is insulated from direct patient input and isolated from patients' online social networks and ever-growing arrays of ubiquitous sensors. Moreover, recent years have seen an explosion in the use of smartphones and tablet computing with connectivity either to the cellular phone network or wirelessly to local area networks, the potential of which for primary care has barely been touched. Future primary care systems will be more integrated with these emerging data sources, thus closer to a true EHR. Table 5.3 lists a range of relevant emerging data sources with some of their key characteristics.

Through mobile technology, healthcare workers or others can make assessments in the community that can contribute to the EHR. For instance, mobile applications have been applied for wound imaging and measurement by community nurses[60] and for community health workers to conduct cardiovascular risk screening.[61] In Japan, postal workers already provide a monitoring service for the elderly, with plans for the wide-scale rollout of a suite of tablet-based health applications for use by the postal workers and the elderly themselves.[62] Indeed, there is now a wide range of health management mobile technologies for direct use by patients – such as applications for asthma management[63] – which creates a wealth of data for integration with the EHR.

Patient computer literacy can be harnessed by providing them with direct access to systems that integrate with the traditional primary care EMR. Online portals provide patients with a Web-based view of their own record, including the ability to have a secure email exchange with their physician.[64] The Electronic Case-Finding and Help Assessment Tool (eCHAT) conducts systematic screening and assesses patient interest in interventions to modify their lifestyle or help with mental health issues.[65] Assessment is completed in the waiting room using a tablet computer and a summary is then waiting for the primary care physician, displayed within the EMR system at the time of consult. Increasingly, patients bring their own hardware to the consult (e.g. smartphones) and could be notified to undertake assessment before arriving at the practice.

Since so many of today's health consumers are active computer users, analysis of large-scale Web search logs can detect regional outbreaks of influenza 7–10 days earlier than conventional public health surveillance systems.[66] Beyond just querying the Web, health consumers participate in structured investigations of drug effectiveness for their personal health situation with the support of social media. PatientsLikeMe is an online community built to support health consumers in sharing information about their treatments, symptoms and outcomes.[67] The PatientsLikeMe system supports users in entering structured treatment history data, including dosages and ratings of side effects and perceived effectiveness. With growing health consumer belief in the effectiveness of patients advising each other (e.g. as promoted by 'e-patient Dave'[68]),

TABLE 5.3 Emerging data sources and their key characteristics

Data source	Who enters the data	What data are provided
Mobile applications	Nurses, community health workers or patients	Monitoring and risk assessments; levels of activity on therapies; progress (e.g. wound size)
Patient portals	Patients (and possibly doctors, nurses or other staff in response)	Patients see select portions of the electronic medical record (e.g. medications and approved lab test results) and can request medication refills and post questions to the primary care staff
Patient online assessment surveys	Patients (in clinic or on their own initiative out of clinic)	Measures of problem severity (e.g. Patient Health Questionnaire 9 [PHQ-9] depression scale)[72] and interest in services to address need
Patient social networks	Patients in discourse with one another	Symptoms and progress; rich natural language discourse on coping strategies; patient-organised 'trials'
Internet of things and home telemonitoring	Sensors log data automatically (or users enter data from display)	Clinical observations (e.g. weight, blood pressure); physical activity monitoring; adherence/compliance monitoring

we can expect patient-contributed data to become an increasingly relevant component of EHR content.

A further emerging data source is the 'Internet of things' (IOT) – the extension of the Internet to the physical world through decreasing cost of sensors and increasing ease of sharing data.[69] Recent developments by IOT start-ups include diapers that test for urinary tract infections and smart pills that signal when they have been ingested by sensing contact with stomach fluid.[70] The concept of 'home telemonitoring' using more conventional sensors (e.g. home blood pressure and glycaemic measurement uploading direct to computer or input by the patient to a portal) has been around for some time. However, monitoring alone is not always effective as an intervention; success is more likely when telemonitoring is combined with caregiver involvement and clinician notification.[71] Further dimensions of the primary care data space will emerge as Internet-based services and IOT sensors become more commonplace and when appropriate technical and ethical frameworks for their linkage to the primary care EHR are established.

SECTION I REFERENCES

1. Loudon I. *Medical Care and the General Practitioner 1750–1850*. Oxford: Clarendon Press, 1986.
2. Thomson A. Westminster Medical Society, November 1, 1828.: Professor Thomson in the chair. *Lancet* 1828; **11**(271): 176–7.
3. Tait I. History of the college. London: Royal College of General Practitioners (RCGP), 2002. Available at: http://www.rcgp.org.uk/about-us/history-heritage-and-archive/history-of-the-college.aspx (accessed 24 November 2015).
4. American Board of General Practice. Welcome to the board. http://www.abgp.org/.
5. Muldoon LK, Hogg WE, Levitt M. Primary care (PC) and primary health care (PHC). What is the difference? *Canadian Journal of Public Health* 2006; **97**(5): 409–11.
6. Fry J, Halser J, editors. *Primary Health Care 2000*. New York: Churchill Livingstone, 1986.
7. World Organization of Family Doctors (WONCA). WONCA in brief. Available at: http://www.globalfamilydoctor.com/AboutWonca/brief.aspx (accessed 24 November 2015).
8. International Conference on Primary Health Care. *Declaration of Alma-Ata: International Conference on Primary Health Care, Alma-Ata, USSR, 6–12 September 1978*. Alma-Ata: World Health Organization, 1978. Available at: http://www.who.int/publications/almaata_declaration_en.pdf (accessed 24 November 2015).
9. Howie JG, Whitefield M, editors. *Academic General Practice in the UK Medical Schools, 1948–2000: A Short History*. Edinburgh: Edinburgh University, 2011.
10. Howie JGR. Academic general practice: reflections on a 60-year journey. *British Journal of General Practice* 2010; **60**(577): 620–3.
11. Goodyear-Smith F. JPHC achieves MEDLINE status. *Journal of Primary Health Care* 2010; **2**(3): 178–9.
12. Beasley JW, Starfield B, van Weel C et al. Global health and primary care research. *Journal of the American Board of Family Medicine* 2007; **20**(6): 518–26.
13. Starfield B. A framework for primary care research. *Journal of Family Practice* 1996; **42**(2): 181–5.
14. Mold JW, Green LA. Primary care research: revisiting its definition and rationale. *Journal of Family Practice* 2000; **49**(3): 206–8.
15. van Weel C, Smith H, Beasley JW. Family practice research networks. Experiences from 3 countries. *Journal of Family Practice* 2000; **49**(10): 938–43.
16. Hahn DL, Golubjatnikov R. Asthma and chlamydial infection: a case series. *Journal of Family Practice* 1994; **38**(6): 589–95.
17. Wetterneck TB, Lapin JA, Krueger DJ et al. Development of a primary care physician task list to evaluate clinic visit workflow. *BMJ Quality & Safety* 2012; **21**(1): 47–53.
18. Starfield B, Shi L, Macinko J. Contribution of primary care to health systems and health. *Milbank Quarterly* 2005; **83**(3): 457–502.
19. Prunuske JP, Deci DM. Learning environment: the impact of clerkship location on instructional quality. *Family Medicine* 2013; **45**(3): 193–6.
20. Donaldson M, Yordy K, Vanselow N. *Defining Primary Care: An Interim Report*. Washington: National Academy Press, 1994.
21. World Health Organization (WHO). *The World Health Report 2008: Primary Health Care; Now More than Ever*. Geneva: WHO, 2008. Available at: http://www.who.int/whr/2008/whr08_en.pdf (accessed 24 November 2015).
22. Beasley J, Karsh B-T. What can we learn from effective collaboration in primary care research? One success story. *Primary Health Care Research & Development* 2010; **11**(3): 203–5.
23. Habermas J. *Knowledge and Human Interests*. Boston: Beacon Press, 1972.

24. Treweek S, Zwarenstein M. Making trials matter: pragmatic and explanatory trials and the problem of applicability. *Trials* 2009; **10**: 37.

25. Van Deventer C, Mash B. African primary care research: quality improvement cycles. *African Journal of Primary Health Care & Family Medicine* 2014; **6**(1): E1–7.

26. Howe A. *Medical Generalism: Why Expertise in Whole Person Medicine Matters.* London: RCGP, 2012.

27. Mash B, Ogunbanjo GA. African primary care research: quantitative analysis and presentation of results. *African Journal of Primary Health Care & Family Medicine* 2014; **6**(1).

28. Reid S, Mash B. African primary care research: qualitative interviewing in primary care. *African Journal of Primary Health Care & Family Medicine* 2014; **6**(1).

29. Mash B. African primary care research: participatory action research. *African Journal of Primary Health Care & Family Medicine* 2014; **6**(1).

30. Nwanze O, Mash R. Evaluation of a project to reduce morbidity and mortality from traditional male circumcision in Umlamli, Eastern Cape, South Africa: outcome mapping. *South African Family Practice* 2012; **54**(3): 237–43.

31. Mash B, Meulenberg-Buskens I. 'Holding it lightly': the co-operative inquiry group: a method for developing educational materials. *Medical Education* 2001; **35**(12): 1108–14.

32. Zuber-Skerritt O. *Action Research in Higher Education: Examples and Reflections.* London: Kogan Page, 1992.

33. Edwards N, Barker PM. The importance of context in implementation research. *Journal of Acquired Immune Deficiency Syndromes* 2014; **67** (Suppl. 2): S157–62.

34. Nilsen P, Ståhl C, Roback K et al. Never the twain shall meet? A comparison of implementation science and policy implementation research. *Implementation Science* 2013; **8**: 63.

35. Jagosh J, Macaulay AC, Pluye P et al. Uncovering the benefits of participatory research: implications of a realist review for health research and practice. *Milbank Quarterly* 2012; **90**(2): 311–46.

36. Janamian T, Jackson C, Dunbar JA. Co-creating value in research: stakeholders' perspectives. *Medical Journal of Australia* 2014; **201**(Suppl. 3): S44–6.

37. ESSENCE on Health Research. *Seven Principles for Strengthening Research Capacity in Low- and Middle-Income Countries: Simple Ideas in a Complex World.* Geneva: Special Programme for Research and Training in Tropical Diseases (TDR) / WHO, 2014. Available at: http://www.who.int/tdr/publications/seven-principles/en/ (accessed 24 November 2015).

38. Mash B, Essuman A, Ratansi R et al. African primary care research: current situation, priorities and capacity building. *African Journal of Primary Health Care & Family Medicine* 2014; **6**(1).

39. De Maeseneer J, van Weel C, Egilman D et al. Strengthening primary care: addressing the disparity between vertical and horizontal investment. *British Journal of General Practice* 2008; **58**(546): 3–4.

40. Macaulay AC, Jagosh J, Seller R et al. Assessing the benefits of participatory research: a rationale for a realist review. *Global Health Promotion* 2011; **18**(2): 45–8.

41. Mathie, E, Wilson P, Poland F et al. Consumer involvement in health research: a UK scoping and survey. *International Journal of Consumer Studies* 2014; **38**(10): 35–44.

42. Furukawa MF, King J, Patel V et al. Despite substantial progress in EHR adoption, health information exchange and patient engagement remain low in office settings. *Health Affairs* 2014; **33**(9): 1672–9.

43. Shoen C, Osborn R, Huynh PT et al. On the front lines of care: primary care doctors' office systems, experiences, and views in seven countries. *Health Affairs* 2006; **25**: w555–71.

44. Marcotte L, Seidman J, Trudel K et al. Achieving meaningful use of health information technology: a guide for physicians to the EHR incentive programs. *Archives of Internal Medicine* 2012; **172**(9): 731–6.

45. McInnes DK, Saltman DC, Kidd MR. General practitioners' use of computers for prescribing and electronic health records: results from a national survey. *Medical Journal of Australia* 2006; **185**(2): 88–91.

46. Akanbi MO, Ocheke AN, Agaba PA et al. Use of electronic health records in sub-Saharan Africa: progress and challenges. *Journal of Medicine in the Tropics* 2012; **14**(1): 1–6.

47. Protti D, Johansen I, Perez-Torres F. Comparing the application of health information technology in primary care in Denmark and Andalucía, Spain. *International Journal of Medical Informatics* 2009; **78**(4): 270–83.

48. WHO. *International Classification of Diseases (ICD-10)*. Geneva: WHO, 2015. Available at: http://www.who.int/classifications/icd/en/ (accessed 24 November 2015).

49. World Organization of Family Doctors (WONCA) International Classification Committee. *International Classification of Primary Care*. Geneva: WHO, 1998.

50. WONCA. WONCA Working Party: WICC (International Classification). Available at: http://www.globalfamilydoctor.com/groups/WorkingParties/wicc.aspx (accessed 24 November 2015).

51. Ohno-Machado L, Nadkarni P, Johnson K. Natural language processing: algorithms and tools to extract computable information from EHRs and from the biomedical literature. *Journal of the American Medical Informatics Association* 2013; **20**(5): 805.

52. Mabotuwana T, Warren J, Harrison J et al. What can primary care prescribing data tell us about individual adherence to long-term medication? Comparison to pharmacy dispensing data. *Pharmacoepidemiology and Drug Safety* 2009; **18**(10): 956–64.

53. Rollman BL, Fischer GS, Zhu F et al. Comparison of electronic physician prompts versus waitroom case-finding on clinical trial enrollment. *Journal of General Internal Medicine* 2008; **23**(4): 447–50.

54. Austin PC. An introduction to propensity score methods for reducing the effects of confounding in observational studies. *Multivariate Behavioral Research* 2011; **46**(3): 399–424.

55. Wennberg JE. Dealing with medical practice variations: a proposal for action. *Health Affairs* 1984; **3**(2): 6–32.

56. Klompas M, McVetta J, Lazarus R et al. Integrating clinical practice and public health surveillance using electronic medical record systems. *American Journal of Public Health* 2012; **102** (Suppl. 3): S325–32.

57. Jin HW, Chen J, He H et al. Mining unexpected temporal associations: applications in detecting adverse drug reactions. *IEEE Transactions on Information Technology in Biomedicine* 2008; **12**(4): 488–500.

58. Office of Civil Rights. Guidance regarding methods for de-identification of protected health information in accordance with the Health Insurance Portability and Accountability Act (HIPAA) privacy rule. Washington DC: US Department of Health and Human Services, 2010. Available at: http://www.hhs.gov/ocr/privacy/hipaa/understanding/coveredentities/De-identification/guidance.html (accessed 24 November 2015).

59. El Emam K. Methods for the de-identification of electronic health records for genomic research. *Genome Medicine* 2011; **3**(4): 25.

60. Miller C, Karimi L, Donohue L et al. Interrater and intrarater reliability of silhouette wound imaging device. *Advances in Skin & Wound Care* 2012; **25**(11): 513–8.

61. Surka S, Edirippulige S, Steyn K et al. Evaluating the use of mobile phone technology to enhance cardiovascular disease screening by community health workers. *International Journal of Medical Informatics* 2014; **83**(9): 648–54.

62. O'Connor F. Apple, IBM to bring iPads to 5 million Japanese seniors. *PCWorld*, 30 April 2015. Available at: http://www.pcworld.com/article/2917332/apple-ibm-to-bring-ipads-to-5-million-japanese-seniors.html (accessed 24 November 2015).

63. Marcano Belisario JS, Huckvale K, Greenfield G et al. Smartphone and tablet self management apps for asthma. *Cochrane Database of Systematic Reviews* 2013; **11**:CD010013.

64. Garrido T, Meng D, Wang JJ et al. Secure e-mailing between physicians and patients: transformational change in ambulatory care. *Journal of Ambulatory Care Management* 2014; **37**(3): 211–18.

65. Goodyear-Smith F, Warren J, Elley CR. The eCHAT program to facilitate healthy changes in New Zealand primary care. *Journal of the American Board of Family Medicine* 2013; **26**(2): 177–82.

66. Carneiro HA, Mylonakis E. Google trends: a web-based tool for real-time surveillance of disease outbreaks. *Clinical Infectious Diseases* 2009; **49**(10): 1557–64.

67. Frost JH, Massagli MP. Social uses of personal health information within PatientsLikeMe, an online patient community: what can happen when patients have access to one another's data. *Journal of Medical Internet Research* 2008; **10**(3): e15.

68. deBronkart D. How the e-patient community helped save my life: an essay by Dave deBronkart. *BMJ* 2013; **346**: f1990.

69. Miorandi D, Sicari S, De Pellegrini F et al. Internet of things: vision, applications and research challenges. *Ad Hoc Networks* 2012; **10**(7): 1497–516.

70. Hamilton L. 4 ways the Internet of things is transforming healthcare. *Forbes*, 26 March 2014. Available at: http://www.forbes.com/sites/85broads/2014/03/26/4-ways-the-internet-of-things-is-transforming-healthcare/ (accessed 24 November 2015).

71. Aikens JE, Rosland AM, Piette JD. Improvements in illness self-management and psychological distress associated with telemonitoring support for adults with diabetes. *Primary Care Diabetes* 2015; **9**(2): 127–34.

72. Kroenke K, Spitzer RL, Williams JB. The PHQ-9: validity of a brief depression severity measure. *Journal of General Internal Medicine* 2001; **16**(9): 606–13.

The contribution of primary care research to health and health systems

Introduction

....

Bob Mash

This section describes the important contribution that primary care research can make to people's health and healthcare. The section takes the typology of primary care research, presented in Section I, as a framework.

The first part of this section, therefore, deals with the contribution of primary care research to clinical care and the management of conditions typically seen. Clinical research has been split up into a number of different perspectives. First, David Mant outlines the contribution of primary care research to new knowledge on how to tackle the burden of disease in terms of disease prevention, early diagnosis, treatment of acute illness and management of chronic conditions. Following on from this, Felicity Goodyear-Smith describes how primary care research can contribute to the translation or implementation of existing knowledge into clinical practice. Carl de Wet then tackles research that focuses on improving quality and patient safety in primary care. Finally, Christos Lionis and Elena Petelos remind us that patient-centredness is at the heart of medical generalism and that primary care research should remain true to this philosophy of whole-person medicine.

In the second part of the section, Dee Mangin looks at the contribution of primary care research to health services. The focus here is on the core dimensions of effective primary care, which cut across all diseases and conditions seen. These include access, first contact care, person-centredness, continuity of care, comprehensiveness and coordination of care. Health services that manage to embody these core dimensions in their ethos and organisation of care have a greater impact on the health of people and can also improve health equity. Linked to this perspective is the contribution of primary care research to strengthening health systems, and Luisa Pettigrew outlines these issues in terms of financing mechanisms, leadership and governance of primary care.

In the final part of this section, Wim Peersman and Jan De Maeseneer discuss the contribution of primary care research to the development of the primary care workforce through education and training. They illustrate their argument by reference to the Human Resources for African Primary Health Care (HURAPRIM) project, which attempted to address the human resources for health crisis in the African continent.

CHAPTER 6

Tackling the burden of disease with primary care research

....

David Mant

Research is not the first thing that comes to mind in tackling anything important like the burden of disease; when facing a long queue of sick people, I don't want the help of a researcher. But, of course, most advances in medicine over the ages have been the results of research. Drugs and vaccines are the most obvious examples, but simple public health measures, from clean drinking water to smoking cessation advice, also reflect careful research into the causes of illness.

The advances in scientific medicine over the past 50 years have tended to over-shadow the importance of applied clinical research, particularly research in primary care. Many aspects of clinical research require access to laboratory facilities, which are more cost-effectively funded in a specialist hospital setting and require a competence in basic science – something now rare in primary care clinicians. So in some countries, the importance of applied clinical research in primary care has been forgotten. But the quality of primary care is still the prime determinant of the outcome and overall cost of healthcare in these countries. And it is impossible to provide high-quality primary care without an evidence base – in other words, without research in primary care.

THE GLOBAL BURDEN OF DISEASE

Clinicians working in the community have one great advantage over their hospital peers – the general nature of their clinical practice gives them a better understanding of the overall burden of disease. The most up-to-date figures come from the Global Burden of Disease (GBD) Study which estimated annual disease-specific mortality rates for 188 countries between 1990 and 2013.[1] The top six diseases in terms of years of life lost in 2013 were: (1) ischaemic heart disease, (2) lower respiratory infections, (3) stroke, (4) diarrhoeal diseases, (5) road injuries, and (6) HIV/AIDS. This ranking reflects an increase since 1990 in the relative importance of the non-communicable diseases (ischaemic heart disease, stroke and road injuries) and a fall in deaths from respiratory and diarrhoeal diseases. Malaria ranks just outside the top six overall (at number eight, the same as in 1990), but it remains in the top five causes of death in children. The most important pathogens remain rotavirus and pneumococcus. The most important cancers are lung (rank 15) followed by liver, stomach, colorectal and breast.

HOW PRIMARY CARE RESEARCH TACKLES THIS BURDEN

Research in primary care makes its impact in one of five ways – by working out how best to: (1) prevent disease, (2) diagnose serious illness at an early and curable stage, (3) treat acute illness effectively before it becomes serious, (4) manage chronic illness to prevent deterioration and acute complications requiring hospital care, and (5) deliver primary care more efficiently and cost-effectively. Research in all five categories can have substantial impact, but only if it addresses an important issue that does reflect the burden of disease and does not stop until the issue is resolved. The best way to demonstrate how this works is to give actual examples, one in each category.

RESEARCH TO PREVENT DISEASE

Research into prevention is a good starting point for primary care researchers wanting to reduce the burden of disease, because activities such as vaccination and supporting smoking cessation are among the most effective interventions you can make in primary care.[2] Securing external support and research funding for prevention is less difficult than for clinical research – hospital clinicians tend to be less interested and less likely to feel that you are stepping on their toes. There are many good examples of large-scale primary care trials,[3,4] as well as primary care–led systematic reviews,[5] of simple preventive interventions that have had global impact.

A key lesson from this research is the importance of focusing primary care effort on secondary rather than primary prevention.[6] However, my personal interest in prevention was, paradoxically, inspired by an example of very effective primary prevention resulting from research done by a general practitioner almost 100 years before my birth. It addressed the problem of cholera (diarrhoeal illness is still the fourth most common cause of global mortality) and is summarised in Box 6.1.[7] It convinced me that undertaking research as a practising clinician in primary care is possible and can have more impact on the burden of disease than just treating illness.

The story outlined in Box 6.1 contains two key lessons for any primary care researcher. The first lesson is to choose a research question that is important, both to you and to the local community. Working as a general practitioner in London, Snow was becoming overwhelmed by the growing number of cases of cholera. He couldn't cope with the workload and his treatments were ineffective – first his cholera patients and then the rest of their families all seemed to die. So he felt he had no option but to try to find out why. His methods were akin to police work, visiting the houses of those who had died and asking questions about the circumstances surrounding each death. He didn't need a laboratory, just painstaking determination, careful record keeping

---

BOX 6.1 An investigation into an outbreak of cholera in London in 1854[7]

Design: Observational research.

Setting: Locality around the clinical practice and home of the investigator (Dr. John Snow) in the Soho district of central London.

Method: Mapping the location of the 578 deaths; conducting qualitative interviews with local residents; subsequent follow-up research to relate annual death rates to source of water supply – analyses stratified by both individual household and residential borough.

Main findings: The map indicated clustering of deaths around one public water pump in Broad Street. The qualitative interviews revealed that deaths in houses some distance from the pump occurred mainly in people who collected water from the pump (because they worked nearby or preferred its taste). Respondents also reported that two groups of local people seemed to be immune from cholera – paupers in the workhouse and brewery workers. The workhouse had its own well. The brewery workers drank ale at work rather than water.

Outcome: The handle of the water pump in Broad Street was removed and the cholera outbreak subsided. Although there remains controversy about the extent to which this was causal, there is no doubt that Snow's follow-up research on the link between water supply and cholera contributed substantially to the decision to prioritise provision of a clean water supply and effective sewerage system in London in the next decade.

---

and the wit to recognise, eventually, that those who hadn't drunk the water from the local pump hadn't got sick.

The second key lesson from the story is that the research itself doesn't change anything. It is widely believed that Snow stopped the cholera epidemic by taking the handle off the local water pump, to popular acclaim. In fact, the epidemic was probably subsiding, because most susceptible people had already died, and as a result there was strong public pressure to replace the pump handle. Snow not only had to face down this opposition but also had to spend considerably more effort in assembling further evidence to convince local politicians that the epidemic would recur if London continued to get its water from shallow wells without constructing an adequate sewerage system. Publishing your findings and being right are not enough to make an impact on the burden of disease.

RESEARCH ON EARLY DIAGNOSIS

Most burdensome diseases are treated more effectively if they are diagnosed at an early stage. The most important determinant of the outcome of cancer is the stage at which it is diagnosed and hence the point at which treatment is started. Speed of diagnosis

---

BOX 6.2 Pre-hospital diagnosis of meningococcal disease in children[8]

Design: Observational study.

Participants and setting: Parents of 448 cases of children (103 fatal, 345 non-fatal) aged under 16 years with meningococcal rash from across the UK.

Method: Data about the course of illness before admission to hospital were obtained from interviews with parents and from primary care records.

Main findings: The time window for clinical diagnosis is narrow. Most children had only non-specific symptoms in the first 4–6 hours, but were close to death by 24 hours. Only 165 (51%) children were sent to hospital after the first consultation. The classic features of haemorrhagic rash, meningism and impaired consciousness developed late (median onset 13–22 hours). By contrast, 72% of children had early symptoms of sepsis (leg pains, cold hands and feet, abnormal skin colour) that first developed at a median time of 8 hours, much earlier than the median time to hospital admission of 19 hours.

Outcome: Revision of clinical guidelines.

---

and treatment is also crucial in determining the outcome of other conditions in the top-six list of globally important problems cited earlier in 'The global burden of disease' subsection – stroke, heart disease and trauma. But the best example of the importance of primary care research to diagnosis is provided not by these conditions but by a study on the diagnosis of meningococcal disease in children, summarised in Box 6.2.[8]

The example given in Box 6.2 exemplifies the importance of carrying out research in primary care. Meningococcal disease develops and kills rapidly, and all previous diagnostic research ignored the evolution of the illness before arrival at the hospital. The fact that all textbooks based their diagnostic advice on symptoms at arrival in hospital contributed substantially to the fact that 50% of cases were being missed when first seen in primary care. The research also highlights the value of effective joint working between hospital specialists and primary care doctors. Further, importantly, the primary care involvement was stimulated by a local problem – delay in the diagnosis of a child with meningococcal disease in my own general practice.

RESEARCH ON TREATING ACUTE ILLNESS

Although research on treating acute illness in primary care is essential, this does not imply that it is essential that the effectiveness of every medicine needs to be trialled in primary care. The effectiveness of a drug used in primary care can often be estimated from a trial done in a hospital population. However, there are exceptions. Some acute illnesses are rarely seen in hospital, so, unless trials are done in primary care, there will be no evidence to guide treatment. Others only ever reach hospital at a late (and therefore much more serious) stage, when the underlying pathology has evolved substantially, so the relative effect of a medicine will not be the same in primary and secondary care. And, of course, drugs are not the only treatment for acute illness – many non-drug treatments (such as surgery) are equally important and very dependent on the skill of the clinician delivering them. The levels of skill, and quality assurance of performance, may vary substantially between primary and secondary care settings.

Lower respiratory infection is still the most important acute illness presenting in primary care contributing to the overall burden of disease, and the Genomics to Combat Resistance against Antibiotics in Community-Acquired LRTI [lower respiratory tract infection] in Europe (GRACE) trial of amoxicillin treatment for lower respiratory symptoms is an extremely good example of how primary care trials can be conducted across international boundaries.[9] The trial recruited over 2000 participants from 12 countries. However, I've chosen instead the example of a trial of a non-drug treatment for respiratory infection – glue ear (otitis media with effusion). This trial is summarised in Box 6.3.[10]

Glue ear is a common childhood problem globally and an important cause of deafness and developmental impairment. Antibiotics have little effect, and surgical treatment (insertion of grommets) is neither very widely available nor affordable in many countries. In contrast, auto-inflation (using a small balloon to blow air into the

---

BOX 6.3 Non-invasive treatment of glue ear in children[10]

Design: Randomised clinical trial.

Participants and setting: A total of 320 children aged 4–11 years with otitis media with effusion drawn from 43 general practices in the UK.

Method: Children were allocated to receive either auto-inflation using a nasal balloon three times daily for 1–3 months plus usual care or usual care alone. Clearance of middle-ear fluid at 1 and 3 months was assessed by experts masked to allocation.

Main findings: Auto-inflation in children is acceptable to children, feasible to teach in primary care and effective both at clearing effusions and improving symptoms and quality of life. Those receiving auto-inflation were more likely than controls to have normal tympanograms at 1 month (47.3% v. 35.6%; adjusted relative risk [RR] 1.36, 95% confidence interval [CI] 0.99 to 1.88) and at 3 months (49.6% v. 38.3%; adjusted RR 1.37, 95% CI 1.03 to 1.83; number needed to treat 9).

Outcome: This is a recent study and its impact will depend on effective global implementation of its findings, but the potential for reducing disease burden and health service costs is substantial (e.g. in the USA in 2004, there were an estimated 2.2 million episodes of glue ear, costing US$4 billion dollars).

child's nostril to clear the Eustachian tube) is an extremely cheap treatment that can be overseen by parents after minimal instruction in primary care.

The importance of the trial described in Box 6.3 stems less from its results – although it showed auto-inflation works, the number needed to treat is quite high – and more from the fact that, before it was done, the non-surgical treatment of children with glue ear in primary care was largely an evidence-free zone.[10] The trial guides everyday care and will avoid children being subjected to unnecessary surgery, and it also has important methodological lessons for primary care researchers. Trials of both drugs and non-drug treatments are only useful if they are done to a high methodological standard – with effective randomisation, blind assessment of objective outcomes and an intention-to-treat analysis based on low loss to follow-up. Without this attention to methodological quality, it isn't possible to believe the results. The trial shows that, even to assess an operator-dependent non-drug intervention, this high level of methodological quality is achievable in primary care on a collaborative basis – it involved 43 separate primary care health centres working closely together. Once again, it shows the value of employing modern technology and collaborating effectively with basic scientists and secondary care in measuring the main outcome accurately and objectively using high-quality tympanometry.

RESEARCH ON MANAGING CHRONIC ILLNESS

The shift in the global burden of disease from infective to non-infective causes was highlighted in the GBD Study cited earlier.[1] This has increased the relative importance of managing chronic illness effectively in primary care, particularly the risk factors for the deterioration of vascular and renal function that cause heart attacks and strokes (such as diabetes, high blood pressure and hyperlipidaemia). Failure to manage these risk factors effectively in primary care not only substantially increases the burden of disease but also the cost and affordability of health services.

There are many studies that could be used as examples here. The first large-scale trial in primary care in the UK (completed in 1985) was the mild hypertension trial which first showed that treating people with a diastolic blood pressure of 90–109 mmHg almost halved the number of people getting strokes.[11] There have subsequently been a number of other impressive primary care trials showing that 'integrated care' (care involving both hospital specialist and primary care practitioners) provides better health outcomes than hospital care alone for both asthma and diabetes.[12,13] However, achieving this aim of integrated care is not easy in practice, and research on how to implement care is equally important. I've therefore chosen as an example a qualitative research study investigating the barriers to effective joint working between primary care clinicians and hospital specialists (Box 6.4).[14]

The value of qualitative research is often overlooked, but it can provide an important reality check, which is often lacking from the results of clinical trials and other quantitative research studies. As was shown in the first example (Box 6.1), finding out what should be done is not enough. To have impact on the burden of disease, you need to

---

BOX 6.4 Qualitative study of the barriers to effective shared care among primary care and hospital doctors[14]

Design: Qualitative study.

Participants and setting: Forty-eight general practitioners and 13 hospital doctors in one region of the UK.

Method: Thematic analysis of semi-structured interviews to investigate how well arrangements for shared care functioned and to identify barriers to effective working, particularly in relation to prescribing.

Main findings: The key themes identified were clinical responsibility, cost-shifting, availability of medicines, clinician satisfaction and the nature of the prescribing relationship. Eight quality indicators were devised to define good practice in the prescribing of medicines when treatment is shared between primary and secondary care.

Outcome: These were preliminary but important findings for policymakers indicating that achieving the benefits of shared care shown in clinical trials needed more than a central edict. It highlighted the interpersonal and organisational issues that need to be addressed before hospital and primary care doctors will work together effectively in practice.

---

effect change – and achieving change requires an in-depth understanding of the current reality, particularly the attitudes and working conditions of those clinicians who will have to implement the change. Qualitative research is a powerful tool in understanding the key issues.

RESEARCH TO AVOID POOR CARE

The quality of primary care can often be constrained by lack of evidence about what should be done. But, much more often, a high disease burden reflects a failure to deliver what we already know. We therefore need research to identify failures to deliver primary care to a high (evidence-based) standard and the reasons for these failures. We also need to assess the effectiveness of different strategies to deal with failure and improve care quality. The qualitative study cited in Box 6.4 is one element of this process, but research on delivering better care encompasses a much wider range of research designs. For example, a narrative review of strategies to improve health worker performance in low-income countries drew attention to a range of clinical trials focusing on interventions in primary care;[15] a recent systematic review identified more than 32 such trials undertaken in sub-Saharan Africa alone.[16] However, it is sometimes necessary for research to ask wider policy questions on how best to deliver care, such as the relative benefits of supply- and demand-led financing and the optimal payment

> **BOX 6.5** Effects of pay-for-performance on the
> quality of primary care in England[17]
>
> **Design:** Observational study.
>
> **Setting:** Forty-two representative general practices in the UK.
>
> **Method:** Interrupted time-series analysis of the quality of care with data collected
> at two time points before implementation of the pay-for-performance scheme (1998
> and 2003) and at two time points after implementation (2005 and 2007). At each time
> point, data on the care of patients with asthma, diabetes or coronary heart disease
> were extracted from medical records; data on patients' perceptions of access to care,
> continuity of care and interpersonal aspects of care were collected from questionnaires.
>
> **Main findings:** Between 2003 and 2005, the rate of improvement in the quality of care
> increased for asthma and diabetes (probability $p < 0.001$) but not for heart disease.
> By 2007, the rate of improvement had slowed for all three conditions ($p < 0.001$), and
> the quality of those aspects of care that were not associated with an incentive had
> declined for patients with asthma or heart disease. No significant changes were seen
> in patients' reports on access to care or on interpersonal aspects of care. Continuity
> of care was reduced after the introduction of the scheme.

mechanism for clinical services. In answering these questions, formal trials are often infeasible and observational methods are the only option. The final example (Box 6.5) chosen shows the potential high impact of such a design if implemented to a high methodological standard.[17]

This very-large-scale observational study in the UK, of the effect of making about 30% of primary care clinicians' pay based on the quality of care they provided, was possible for two reasons: (1) the researchers worked closely with the government health services responsible for implementing the scheme, adopting a methodology and timescale acceptable to them; and (2) all the clinical records were electronic, allowing care quality to be audited routinely at affordable cost. It is possible to undertake effective clinical audit with paper records, but the advances in IT that have made electronic record keeping possible at affordable cost provide a major new opportunity for large-scale research into primary care quality (see Chapter 5).

CONCLUSION

It is impossible to provide a detailed guide in a short chapter on how to undertake research in primary care that affects the global burden of disease. The examples cited herein are given to inspire and as an illustration of what is possible. The original papers are mostly free on the Internet and are all worth reading. They all address an issue that was both personally important to their authors and had the potential to impact on clinical practice, thereby reducing the global burden of disease. They emphasise the value of aiming high and not wasting time undertaking research that does not address an important question.

As the target readership of this book is global, I was tempted to focus the examples on research undertaken in low-income countries where the disease burden is highest. However, this would have narrowed substantially the choice of examples and suggested that the underlying issues are not global. Undertaking primary care research, like delivering primary care, is much more difficult in countries with limited resources and political instability. But the principles of research methodology – how to undertake research that provides a believable answer – are global and fairly stable over time. Three of the examples given illustrate the benefits of collaboration with experts, both internationally and in the hospital sector. Primary care research to address important global health issues is not something to attempt alone without expert help, even if you have the ability and unquenchable energy of Dr. John Snow. The one very good aspect of the primary care research environment internationally is the willingness of others to be collaborative and supportive.

Research is not an end in itself. For me, the only point of undertaking research in primary care is to improve the quality of care we provide. This means collecting research evidence in order to act on it. And this is the rub – acting on research evidence is context specific. The key question in taking action to implement evidence is less 'What does work?' but more 'What do I have to do locally to make it work?' The challenge for researchers in low- and middle-income countries, particularly in primary care, is to conduct research to provide the necessary evidence about local context to ensure that what we already know can be implemented effectively. Without effective implementation of findings, primary care research will have no impact on the global burden of disease.

CHAPTER 7

How primary care research blends with evidence-based medicine to assist with translation and implementation of evidence into practice

....

Felicity Goodyear-Smith

THE DEVELOPMENT OF EVIDENCE-BASED MEDICINE

In the 1980s, David Sackett, a professor of medicine at McMaster University, Canada, published a series of articles on how to critically appraise medical research to inform safe and effective clinical practice.[18] This work was extended by his colleague Gordon Guyatt in the 1990s, who coined the term 'evidence-based medicine' – clinical practice based on what has been scientifically shown to work for patient management of different conditions.[19] There followed a series of papers in *JAMA* titled 'Users' guides to the medical literature', with a particular focus on interpreting the results of clinical studies and on deciding how to apply these in patient care.[20]

At the same time, Scottish doctor Archibald Cochrane was advocating for the use of randomised controlled trials (RCTs) to improve the effectiveness and efficiency of medical practice. The Cochrane Centre was established in Oxford, England, in 1992 under the leadership of a health services researcher, Iain Chalmers. The aim of the centre was to review and assess the entire body of literature on all interventions. This led to the establishment of the international Cochrane Collaboration in 1993, producing up-to-date systematic reviews and meta-analyses of relevant RCTs of healthcare, and, subsequently, the Cochrane Library database.[21]

Chalmers and Muir Gray, a public health physician, established the Centre for Evidence-Based Medicine in Oxford in 1995, with David Sackett as director. This facilitated the spread of evidence-based medicine to the UK, Europe and beyond.[22]

Clinical practice could now be based on examination of the current evidence rather than tradition or authority.

EVIDENCE-BASED GUIDELINES

By the turn of the century, this evidence was being incorporated into clinical guidelines, directing decisions regarding diagnosis and management in specific areas of health-care. Guidelines usually include consensus statements of what is considered to be best practice and often algorithms to aid decision-making. There was a rapid proliferation of guidelines for a huge variety of conditions – produced regionally, nationally and internationally by professional bodies, healthcare organisations, governments and international collaborations – to help standardise and improve the quality of care. Guidelines rapidly became commonplace.

However, guidelines themselves could be variable in their scientific validity, reliability and usability. In 2002, an international group of researchers from 13 countries (the Appraisal of Guidelines, Research and Evaluation [AGREE] Collaboration) developed and validated a generic tool to appraise the quality of clinical guidelines.[23] This led in turn to the establishment of the Guidelines International Network, with member organisations – such as the UK National Institute for Health and Clinical Excellence (NICE) and the US National Guideline Clearinghouse – applying the AGREE standardised methods to produce quality guidelines.

There has been an exponential increase in the publication of RCTs, systematic reviews distilling the accumulating evidence and guidelines to inform best practice. Increasingly, general practitioners (GPs) are expected to use guidelines to direct their clinical decision-making. In 2004, the Quality and Outcomes Framework (QOF) was introduced in the UK as a pay-for-performance scheme, covering a wide range of clinical and organisational outcomes, with financial rewards for meeting determined targets for these QOF indicators.

As the stack of guidelines accumulated on the consultation room floor, increased effort went into the implementation of guidelines, now a research topic in its own right. Approaches included educational sessions, making summaries available on GPs' computer desktops and algorithms electronically incorporated into clinical pathways.

BENEFITS AND UNINTENDED CONSEQUENCES OF GUIDELINES

There is no doubt that understanding and applying robust scientific evidence from well-conducted trials can improve patient care and health outcomes. For example, achieving quality targets may result in significant health gains among patients with cardiovascular disease.[24]

However, there is also the danger that guidelines can lead to 'cookbook medicine', with less of a holistic, biopsychosocial approach to patient care. Many guidelines synthesise hospital-based studies of homogenous patient groups. This may lead to fragmentation and consequent poor coordination of care. Applying single disease guidelines to a patient with multi-morbidity may lead to polypharmacy and adverse medication interactions. Insufficient resources for all GPs to implement the evidence may increase health disparities. The QOF tick-box approach focuses on what is easy to measure, rather than the less tangible clinical elements such as the nature of the doctor–patient relationship. Population health objectives may conflict with a patient-centred approach to individual care. Consultations have a finite capacity, and the quality of care may reduce for conditions not included in the incentive framework.

BEST PRACTICE REQUIRES SYNTHESIS OF EMPIRICAL AND CONTEXTUAL EVIDENCE

Best practice requires the synthesis of scientific knowledge, the context in which it is applied and 'phronesis' – the accumulated wisdom of the practitioner.[25] Empirical evidence contributes to management decisions made by doctors and their patients but cannot supplant the contextual knowledge that both contribute.

Sackett himself warned that scientific evidence can inform but never replace clinical expertise.[26] Clinical decisions must always involve our patients within the complex and uncertain reality of their lives. Decisions must take into account a large array of factors, including patient preferences; social, moral and legal issues; and resource constraints.

Traditional research has addressed the efficacy (*Can it work?*), effectiveness (*Does it work in practice?*) and efficiency (*Is it worth it?*) of interventions. The gold standard is the RCT using a standardised protocol and heterogeneity of participants minimised to reduce complexity and 'noise' and hence enable generalisability. Typically, measures of determinants are individual attributes such as demographic characteristics. However, these findings may not be applicable to patients in the community whose context is different from study participants, for example, who have multi-morbidities or for who there are resource restraints to receiving the 'ideal' treatment.

IMPLEMENTATION SCIENCE, PARTICIPATORY RESEARCH AND KNOWLEDGE TRANSLATION

The need to address context has led to the growth of implementation science, which seeks to assess dynamic programmes of population health that can adjust to changes in context in real time.[27] Implementation science looks at what works, under which situations and for who, and focuses on interventions that can be adapted to fit and scaled up to enable equitable access. Conducting such research requires a mixed method approach of data collection and study design and an interdisciplinary approach.

Interventions need to have contextual fit, to be responsive to the community and the participants they serve. Implementation science therefore requires co-partnerships between researchers and stakeholders – those people affected by the study issue and/ or responsible for implementing it.[28] Participatory research may involve patients, healthcare providers, health service and health system managers, and policymakers. This adds further challenges and complexity – with respect to heterogeneity of research questions, methods and study designs – to the development and management of a variety of relationships and to the generation of numerous short- and long-term outcomes.

Knowledge translation is required to move knowledge into action. This requires diffusion and dissemination of an innovation and its adoption, as well as the readiness of the system to accept change. Research needs to be ongoing to refine and improve interventions for continuing contextual adaption. Chambers et al. propose a dynamic sustainability framework 'involving continued learning and problem solving, ongoing adaptation of interventions with a primary focus on fit between interventions and multi-level contexts, and expectations for ongoing improvement as opposed to diminishing outcomes over time'.[29] Both positive and unintended negative consequences must be identified through evaluation then fed back for effective and sustained organisational transformation.[30]

SUMMARY

Findings from RCTs will not always be fit for purpose, either in the context of specific patients' care or across a complex health system. Implementation science attempts to provide research-based evidence to identify and implement best practice for people and for populations.

While affordable and life-saving interventions may exist, knowledge may be lacking on how to deliver these across a range of health systems in a diversity of settings. Research needs to be directed at answering questions asked by people working in the real world, rather than those primarily of interest to researchers.[31] Co-creation and collaboration are required.

Implementation research can bridge the gap between what can be achieved in theory and what happens in practice and is being embraced as the means to contextualise empirical science. The field of primary care–based implementation science is growing fast, with the aim of maximising the benefits of health interventions and moving research into practice and policy.

CHAPTER 8

How primary care research contributes to improving the quality and safety of healthcare

....

Carl de Wet

INTRODUCTION

The phrase 'first, do no harm' has been a fundamental principle of healthcare for hundreds, if not thousands, of years. It succinctly describes the duty of clinicians to fulfil the reasonable desire of any patient to receive care that is safe and of high quality. However, a series of landmark studies and reports around the turn of the century provided irrefutable evidence that a significant minority of patients suffers preventable iatrogenic harm during their interactions with healthcare systems.[32-34] This finding has since been replicated by a large number of studies worldwide.[35-37]

The responses to the reported deficiencies in the quality and safety of healthcare have varied considerably. There are those who deny that there is a problem at all, while others acknowledge it and have started taking steps to improve the safety and quality of the care provided by their own units and organisations. In some countries, the safety of patients has been formally recognised and prioritised at a national level, with allocation of additional resources to help solve the problem. For example, Scotland implemented the Scottish Patient Safety Programme in January 2008 with the ambitious aim to measurably improve the safety of care in acute hospitals over a 5-year period. The programme has since been extended and now also includes mental health and primary care.[38]

However, despite more than a decade of growing interest and investments to improve patient safety in many countries, there is still little evidence of widespread reductions in patient harm.[39] What we have learned, though, is that sustained improvements in care quality and safety are facilitated (or hindered) by at least four important factors:[40,41] (1) the availability of adequate and appropriate resources; (2) supportive and visible senior leadership; (3) clinician engagement in and 'ownership' of improvement efforts; and (4) evidence-based interventions that are acceptable, feasible and that produce visible and measurable results. There is another factor that underpins all of the others, yet hasn't always been as explicitly acknowledged – research.

The aims of this chapter are therefore to describe why research – specifically, primary care research (PCR) – is essential to help improve the quality and safety of healthcare and to consider how it fulfils this important role. In the first and largest part of the chapter, the primary contribution of PCR is discussed – namely, the generation of new and useful knowledge. The chapter concludes with a brief reflection about potential secondary contributions of PCR and its synergy with quality improvement (QI).

RESEARCH GENERATES NEW AND USEFUL KNOWLEDGE

Research can be defined as 'a systematic investigation, including research development, testing and evaluation, designed to develop or contribute to generalizable knowledge'.[42] In other words, the main purpose – and value – of research is the *systematic generation* of *new knowledge* that is useful.

The vast majority of all the different types of 'new knowledge' that PCR creates about healthcare quality and safety can be classified into three interlinked groups, depending on whether it relates to: (1) increasing our understanding of the nature and scale of safety and quality deficiencies, (2) improvement interventions and initiatives, or (3) normalising improvement. Each of these three groups is discussed in more detail following.

Group one: primary care research knowledge increases our understanding of care quality and safety

The first group of knowledge includes all the types of information that help us better understand the nature and scale of patient safety and care quality deficiencies. This includes epidemiological studies about the prevalence, incidence and aetiology of patient safety incidents. It also includes the research to create taxonomies, agree the terminology of the disciplines and build their underpinning theories. Due to space constraints, only a small selection of studies will be listed for illustrative purposes.

Several large-scale epidemiological studies to reliably quantify the harm rate in primary care are currently underway and their results are eagerly anticipated. However, because of PCR, we already know that medical errors are relatively common in primary care settings worldwide and that a substantial minority results in preventable harm to patients.[43,44] Consider the following two from the many potential practical examples of PCR studies: (1) it has been estimated that preventable adverse events originating in outpatient settings result in ±75 000 hospital admissions per year in the USA,[45] and (2) that the error rate in primary care in the UK may be 75.6 errors per 1000 consultations.[46]

It is because of PCR that our understanding of the different types of primary care errors, their incidence, antecedent factors and their clinical impact has greatly increased. Of these, medication error has arguably been studied the most. In the UK, Garfield et al. were the first to map out the complete primary care medicines management system.[47] Their systematic review of the evidence of cumulative medication errors in the system found errors in every stage, with error rates often exceeding 50%. Consequently, a minority of patients achieved 'optimum benefit' from their medication. This finding does not only apply to the UK as, irrespective of the country of origin, adverse drug events (ADEs) may affect one in five patients.[48,49]

PCR has revealed that ADEs are usually caused by 'complex and multifaceted' errors, including drug–drug interactions, discrepancies between prescribed and administered drugs, and communication failures.[50,51] A handful of medications – anticoagulant, cardiovascular and non-steroidal anti-inflammatory drugs – are associated with the majority of ADEs.[52] Conversely, if some drugs are not prescribed this may also lead to preventable hospital admissions – for example, anti-anginals and asthma preventers.[53] We now know the risk factors for ADEs include older age, female gender, multiple prescription items, number of daily doses, multi-morbidity, high consultation rates and discrepancies between recorded and actual medication use.[54-56] Similarly, PCR has increased our knowledge about the other error types, such as diagnostic,[57,58] investigation[59,60] and interface errors.[61]

PCR, through generation of this first group of knowledge, contributes to the improvement of care safety and quality in at least four different ways:

1. *PCR helps to justify allocation of resources and improvement efforts.*
   Understanding the nature and scale of a problem is a prerequisite for planning and preparing the actions required to address it. By providing sufficient, reliable evidence of significant and systemic shortfalls in the safety and quality of care, PCR provides the rationale and justification for policymakers and managers to allocate additional resources to help address deficiencies in care quality and safety. The knowledge is also useful to help raise awareness of the need for improving care quality and safety among clinical and non-clinical staff groups, motivate them to participate in improvement initiatives and justify their investment of time and effort as being worthwhile.

2. *PCR helps to inform improvement priorities.*
   Once agreement has been reached that action is justified to address an identified and important problem, it is important to consider how best to direct limited resources. There isn't a single best answer, but it is helpful to consider which aspects of care quality and safety are most amenable to intervention and what type of errors is particularly prevalent or causes significantly more suffering than others. PCR helps to answer these questions.

3. *PCR creates a shared understanding of problems, terminology and taxonomies.*
   An agreed terminology has a number of potential benefits. It helps to reduce unnecessary duplication of research, allows direct comparison and generalisation between settings and enables effective communication about quality and safety of care. Early quality and safety research abounded with a plethora of different terms or the same

terms used to imply different meanings.[62] PCR has helped to prune back the verbal foliage and continues to facilitate the development of a common terminology.[63]

Taxonomies are useful because they facilitate recognition of differences and similarities. More specifically, they provide explanatory power by defining and identifying contributory factors to patient safety and may help facilitate error reporting and aid development of interventions to prevent errors. Dovey et al.[64] and Makeham et al.[65] were among the first to develop taxonomies of primary care medical errors more than a decade ago in the USA and Australia, respectively. Since then, several safety-related taxonomies have been developed and validated for primary care settings in Canada,[66] the UK[46] and New Zealand,[67] among others.

4. *PCR identifies quality and safety performance baselines.*
   Quantifying the quality and safety of care for a specific setting and point in time allows comparison with subsequent, serial measures. Once certain statistical provisos are satisfied,[68] this helps stakeholders to set specific improvement targets, monitor progress and identify when their aims have been achieved.

Group two: primary care research generates knowledge about improvement interventions

The second group of knowledge PCR generates is about improvement interventions, tools, methods and initiatives. This group increases our understanding of how to address deficiencies in care quality and safety. It includes all of the research processes required to produce evidence-based interventions that are feasible, acceptable and useful.

This may require adapting interventions, tools or methods from safety-critical industries and other healthcare settings for primary care. It is an approach that is commonly used in PCR and there are many potential examples, including: (1) the development and testing of a number of validated instruments to measure perceptions of safety culture and climate in primary care settings,[69-71] (2) application of the 'care bundle' approach to improve chronic disease management and as a composite measure of care quality,[72] (3) the development of a preliminary list of 'never events' that are specific to general practice,[73] and (4) extending Trigger Tools application from a metric applied only by external reviewers to a metric used by a wide range of primary care clinicians who could apply the Trigger Review Method to their own patient's medical records in order to detect and learn from latent patient safety incidents and further improve the quality and safety of the care they deliver.[74]

Alternatively, interventions and initiatives can be designed and developed de novo or in collaboration with other agencies. For example, significant event analysis (SEA) is a well-established safety improvement intervention that was developed in UK primary care.[75] General practice teams apply the method to investigate and learn from suboptimal care or other issues of significance that they have identified. Another example is the list of 'always events' for general practice that was recently developed through collaboration between PCR and patients.[76]

Until recently, the majority of PCR activity in the disciplines of patient safety and quality improvement has been aimed at producing group-one types of knowledge.

While a number of potential interventions, tools and methods are now available,[77] there is still a relative paucity of research about their effectiveness or of formal *initiatives* to measurably improve safety or mitigate error in any healthcare setting and particularly in primary care.[78] It was appropriate to focus initial research efforts on generating group-one knowledge, because effective interventions could more readily be produced once there was agreement, understanding and prioritising of a problem. However, there is now an increasingly urgent call for the focus in PCR to shift from description and measurement to improvement.[79]

Several different safety and quality improvement initiatives have been piloted already. Examples include pharmacist-led medication reviews and reconciliation, chronic disease nurse-led protocol management, education programmes for general practitioners and 'complex' interventions to reduce falls in elderly patients.[80,81] There is 'weak evidence to indicate' that pharmacist-led review may reduce medication-related hospital admissions and that eliciting and addressing patients' medication symptoms may help to reduce ADEs.[82,83] However, a meta-analysis of primary care studies found no conclusive evidence that any of these initiatives significantly improved patient safety.[84]

There is some evidence of existing, informal improvement activities intrinsic to primary care settings. For example, an ethnographic case study of UK general practices found that receptionists and administrative staff 'make important "hidden contributions" to quality and safety in repeat prescribing'.[85] Another example is the potential value of mitigation in preventing errors from resulting in patient harm.[86] All healthcare staff and patients and their families are potential mitigators and it has been estimated they may stop up to a fifth of all errors.[87]

There are at least two important benefits from this second group of knowledge created through PCR. The first is that it provides the necessary evidence-based tools, methods and interventions to help improve the quality and safety of primary care. The second benefit is that ineffective interventions are identified and can therefore be discontinued or adapted, thereby sparing precious and limited resources. The history of healthcare is littered with examples of interventions with high initial face-validity that were launched with great expectation only to produce little benefit or, paradoxically, harm to patients. The value of PCR is therefore in either helping to bridge the gap between apparent logic and reality or, alternatively, providing evidence that no bridge exists or can be built.

Group three: primary care research generates knowledge about the normalisation of improvement

The third group of knowledge PCR generates relates to the normalisation of improvement. Normalisation includes all of the required work to implement interventions and initiatives, to spread them within units or organisations and to sustain improvement long enough for it to become embedded and integrated into routine care. These processes are particularly suited to study designs that use conceptual frameworks based on normalisation process theory (NPT).[88] NPT was developed, refined and tested in

UK primary care during the last decade and is therefore particularly suitable for PCR aiming to identify the factors that facilitate or hinder improvement efforts.[89]

Knowledge about the normalisation of improvement in primary care continues to increase, with learning and experiences being reported from many countries worldwide, including Australia,[90] Mexico,[91] South Africa,[92] the Netherlands[93] and the UK.[94] However, the evidence base is still substantially smaller compared with those of the other two groups of knowledge generated through PCR. This is understandable, as normalisation first requires identifying a problem, then the ready availability of suitable interventions to address the problem before longer-term effects can be measured and studied.

What little evidence there is suggests that improvement initiatives driven by clinicians and patients may be more likely to become normalised than those by managers and policies. Unfortunately, there are many challenges in engaging clinicians in quality and safety improvement.[95] One potential solution may be for practical, individualised QI projects to be incorporated into appraisal and revalidation of primary care clinicians.[96] The potential value of PCR is therefore to provide evidence of and explain what works, what doesn't and why.

THE SYNERGISM BETWEEN PRIMARY CARE RESEARCH AND QUALITY IMPROVEMENT

The terms 'quality improvement' and 'research' are often used interchangeably, even by their practitioners. The debate about the nature of their differences has quietened down in recent years, but, from the perspective of considering what the value of PCR may be, it is still worthwhile to acknowledge at least two. The first difference is that QI is considered to be an activity where existing knowledge is applied to a problem that has already been identified in a specific healthcare setting or population and the express aim is to improve care quality and safety.

In reality, many of the core skills that are required to perform effective PCR are equally important and necessary for QI. For example, the ability to clearly formulate a problem (or hypothesis), systematically collect data, to analyse and interpret it correctly by using appropriate statistical methods and to present the findings in a clear and accessible manner to different stakeholders are integral to the success of both QI and PCR. In addition, these tasks often have to be completed within significant budgetary and time constraints and therefore require leadership, management and administrative skills. In other words, many PCR skills, methods and experiences are 'generic' and imminently transferable to other sectors and tasks, including healthcare and QI.

Second, many healthcare systems now routinely collect, aggregate, analyse and learn from their own patient-level data. Clinicians are encouraged to make decisions guided by knowledge produced from this structured learning in combination with the best available evidence. In contrast, there is usually no obligation on frontline staff or healthcare organisations to routinely engage with research, and researchers (in general) are often external to the systems they study.

Another potential strength of PCR is that researchers often have clinical experience or ongoing clinical commitments that provide them not only with unique insights about the quality and safety of their care and the practical challenges to further improve it but also opportunities to implement research and translate research findings into practice. Given that the vast majority of healthcare is delivered in primary care settings,[97] the potential impact of PCR on the quality and safety of care could be huge.

However, the degree to which PCR contributes to QI efforts depends on several factors,[98] including (1) willingness and opportunities for collaboration between researchers, clinicians, patients and quality improvement practitioners; (2) allocation of adequate and appropriate resources; (3) training and support of research and clinical staff; (4) identifying and systemically addressing existing research gaps in primary care; and (5) acknowledging that the quality and safety of care is a priority through word *and* deed.

CONCLUSION

The main contribution of PCR to improving the quality and safety of healthcare is through the systematic generation of new, generalisable knowledge. In this chapter, three main groups of knowledge and the potential value of each were discussed. The first and largest group of knowledge consists of all the types of information that increases our understanding of the nature and scale of problems in healthcare. The second group is all the knowledge about interventions, tools, methods and initiatives to improve care. The third, and currently smallest, group of knowledge is about normalising improvement. A secondary contribution of PCR is in synergy with QI through the transferability of PCR and researchers' skills, methods and experiences.

CHAPTER 9

Making healthcare more person-centred: how primary care research can help bring in the human and patient perspective

....

Christos Lionis and Elena Petelos

INTRODUCTION

Over the last few decades, numerous discussions have focused on primary healthcare (PHC) and primary care research (PCR). Nevertheless, much ambiguity remains as to how the purpose and conduct of PCR may differ from research conducted in other disciplines and settings.

An editorial in *The Lancet* argued that primary care research has experienced a loss of direction and confidence as it tries to define itself.[99] Generating questions about the extent to which PCR may differ, it attempted to explore differences in research conducted in primary care versus other specialised research. The answer is not simple, as we should examine PCR in terms of its potential and actual societal impact, the methodological challenges, the scientific evidence it attempts to generate and the outcomes and associated cost. It is not possible to address all these issues here, but we aim to highlight PCR by focusing on some of the 'right' questions to ask.

We explore the degree to which PCR can focus on patient-centredness and compassion as core attributes of effective primary care. The ultimate aim is to determine how research findings could be utilised for decision-making and to improve PHC delivery and outcomes. The overall focus should be on what has been recently referred to as 'citizen-centred' or 'person-centred' healthcare systems, with involvement of the people independently of their health status in the development and implementation of both research and policy and, ultimately, with active involvement in generating research and policy topics through collaborative stakeholder consultations.

In the past, we had a doctor-centred approach, where the patient was more passive. The era of globalised information and research into the overall quality of care has shown that patients can contribute ideas to improve their treatment and care and their overall experience. In addition, an ageing population and increased life expectancy have been coupled with an exacerbation of chronic illness and multi-morbidity, thus necessitating a new approach to tackling such challenges. A lack of access to personalised care and the failure to care for people have led to a growing dialogue on compassionate care. This has highlighted the need for more exploration of patient-centred care together with the notion of compassion.[100]

Patients with chronic diseases can be empowered to self-manage and improve their adherence to shared management goals, with more effective use of resources in a heavily burdened care system. Research is required into how to incorporate concerns for such patient-centredness into research that assesses health services and the education of health workers, as current approaches are not sufficient to embed this element. This has to start with basic research to develop the tools we need to measure patient-centredness and extend to the selection of relevant health system indicators. Such tools and indicators should also be included in the design of studies that use large clinical data sets and in observational studies. Attention to the context of research findings, engagement with patients to bring to the fore research themes of relevance and a substantial exploration of the concept of patient-centred care through a more humanistic and compassionate lens may all be needed.

PATIENT-CENTRED CARE: A CURRENT FOCUS ACROSS CONTINENTS

The World Health Organization (WHO), in its report on PHC,[101] introduced a clear and supportive framework that emphasised four broad and interlinked policy reforms to address universal coverage, people-centred services, community-oriented primary care and leadership. This has led to a resurgence of interest in people-centred care and a discussion on research into such models of care within the European General Practice Research Network. This has led to the development of the Research Agenda for the European General Practitioner, which captures the evidence relating to the core competencies and characteristics of the World Organization of Family Doctors (WONCA) Europe definition of general practice / family medicine (GP/FM). Its main purpose is to assist both researchers and policymakers to identify and bridge gaps on existing evidence, highlight relevant research topics informed by patient experiences[102] and foster cross-border research collaboration. To inform this effort, a review of the literature was conducted on these core competencies using the concepts of 'person-centred care', 'comprehensive approach' and 'holistic approach'. The review underlined the need to develop and utilise validated instruments to measure these competencies: 'Primary care evolves towards more interdisciplinary care, and research should focus more on the core competency of person-centred team care. There is an urgent need to develop clear definitions and appropriate research instruments for this domain. It will be a particular challenge to study comprehensive approaches in primary-care patients with multimorbidity'.[103]

Patient-centredness is a concept that implies eliciting and understanding patient ideas and preferences. However, little is known about eliciting patient preferences when multiple trade-offs and treatment burdens complicate the decision. This becomes even more relevant when care involves other family members, friends or relatives, and when emotional or psychological issues are prominent.[104] The current global research focus is mostly disease specific and fails to address issues of multi-morbidity, goal-oriented care and patient-centredness in a PHC context.

Effective collaboration between physicians, patients and their families requires a commitment to a compassionate relationship. This requires a primary care provider who is well trained in empathy and effective communication, although there are concerns regarding the extent to which compassion can be taught. Such training is clearly lacking in many settings and in most countries, although a few examples do exist.[105] Increased mobility and migration of patients within and between countries has made the challenge of bridging language and culture for the family physician more common. At the same time, the family physician has new tools and opportunities to explore, such as electronic medical records, Internet resources and new technologies. The management of resources is also increasingly complex, with financial constraints, increased therapeutic options and an ageing population. All of this necessitates the need for continuous professional development.

Institutions have transformed, and new ways of living (urban and semi-urban) have radically modified the needs and options available, creating new gaps for general practitioners (GPs) to bridge, but, also, providing new tools and opportunities to explore, thus necessitating continuous education and improvement and a radical focus shift, along with a need for reallocation of resources.

HOW CAN THE CONTENT OF PRIMARY CARE RESEARCH BE MADE MORE PATIENT-CENTRED, INTEGRATED AND COMPASSIONATE?

The term 'integrated care' has received a lot of attention in the literature, and it is highly relevant to the term 'patient-centred care'. For the term 'integration', we shall co-opt the WHO definition: '[The] management and delivery of health services so that the client receives a continuum of preventive and curative services according to the needs over time and across different levels of the health system'.[106]

Two additional concepts that have received attention and are very relevant to patient-centred and integrated care are 'compassionate care' and 'multi-morbidity'.

Although many authors support the strong link between patient-centred and compassionate care, the Institute of Medicine's (IOM) current definition of 'patient-centred care' has been criticised for lacking an explicit emphasis on compassion.[107] The concept of 'compassionate care' has not attracted the degree of attention it should from the primary care community, as elaborated in *Providing Compassionate Health Care*: 'we can assume that compassion may incorporate other concepts frequently utilized in

FM/GP including patient centeredness and empathy. However, there is still much room for GPs to place more emphasis on non-pharmacological treatment and to emphasize a crossroad of medicine with other disciplines, particularly the psychological and social sciences'.[108] It is has been reported that compassion as a feature of clinical care is decreasing,[109] and that multidisciplinary research needs to explore the relationship between compassionate care and clinical effectiveness and quality.

'Multi-morbidity' pertains to the management in individuals of two or more health conditions simultaneously.[110] Multi-morbidity is often a problem of ageing and increasing frailty, although frailty is more of a clinical syndrome than a disease. Elderly people present an increased risk for poor health outcomes including falls, disability, hospitalisation and mortality.[111,112] Effective management of multi-morbidity requires integrated care, and this becomes even more apparent when mental illness intersects with multi-morbidity.

Langan and colleagues recognise that: 'The central role of mental illness within the multimorbidity continuum [...] invite[s] psychiatrists, GPs, researchers and policy makers urgently to discuss how best to develop and evaluate services that will improve physical, psychological and social outcomes'.[113] In a similar direction, Akner underlines: 'An important challenge for future research and development regarding the management of frailty and multimorbidity in elderly patients is to shift the focus from managing isolated diseases to managing multiple health problems and to expand the traditional medical organ-based examination and treatment with regularly recurring analyses of various system and functional domains'.[114]

INVOLVING THE PATIENT IN THE DEVELOPMENT AND IMPLEMENTATION OF RESEARCH AND POLICY: PATIENT AND PUBLIC INVOLVEMENT IN RESEARCH

All of this is rhetoric without the involvement of the patient in the evaluation of healthcare services and the design and execution of research. The Agency for Healthcare Research and Quality, in its brief report *The Patient-Centered Medical Home: Strategies to put Patients at the Centre of Primary Care*,[115] proposes and emphasises as a key strategy the need for policymakers to engage the patient, actively involving citizens in quality improvement. This essentially means that primary care providers should invite either the patients themselves or the patients' organisations to report their wishes, preferences and perspectives and to assess the quality of their care services. The research design, research feasibility and evaluation processes need to reflect this approach.

The term 'patient and public involvement' (PPI), which promotes 'research being carried out "with" or "by" members of the public rather than "to", "about" or "for" them', has permeated recent development in the UK policy.[116] The UK Department of Health[117] has recommended that PPI should be included in all stages of the review process. However, this is a challenging field, and it is still unknown to what extent the patients or their representatives are or can be involved in the design of research in primary care. It is expected that PPI may contribute to the desired goal of more patient-centred and compassionate care and research. A key aspect of the six core components that WONCA Europe included in their definition of general practice is community orientation. This is directly linked to community engagement which WHO defines as 'a process by which people are enabled to become actively and genuinely involved in defining the issues of concern to them, in making decisions about factors that affect their lives, in formulating and implementing policies, in planning, developing and delivering services and in taking action to achieve change'.[118]

How can we enhance patient engagement not only in self-care but also in patient-centred outcome research, and how can we help patients and the public to make informed healthcare decisions and improve healthcare delivery and outcomes?

The focus of clinical practice and PCR is ultimately the patient or person, with a mission to maintain their health and overall well-being. There are many ways to achieve this objective, but the main one is to assist the patient to make informed decisions through shared decision-making. However, both patient-centred and integrated care have to be examined in terms of the ability of patients to adapt behaviour, modify habits and to self-manage. This idea gives a new direction to approaching the patient, to defining the orientation towards which healthcare services should direct efforts and about how we should measure effectiveness.

Across the world, patients are frequently in a labyrinth of options, frequently confused by contradicting, inadequate or inaccurate information found on the Internet or stemming from multiple consultations with a variety of providers and/or from discussions with friends, family, colleagues or their wider social circle. On the other hand, providers need the capacity and skills to navigate and identify robust evidence for both patients and caregivers and to provide interpretive hints allowing them to process this information, ultimately engaging in shared decision-making that generates an informed healthcare decision. Providers need to translate research findings into a set of options to be offered to their patients, and, ideally, provide them with a toolkit to filter information that may confuse or confound patients even after the initial decision has been made. This is the bridge between clinical practice and research, a continuum and cycle clearly visible in PCR.

The same principles apply to research. Practitioners should not view research as a domain outside their remit but as part of daily practice. Patients should, also, be considered active participants in research, with practitioners engaging and encouraging them to actively participate. For example, practitioners should inform their patients about participation options, either in terms of direct participation or in terms of observing and/or engaging in community initiatives, and should realise this should become part of their daily practice.

It is important to note that, increasingly, the effectiveness of an intervention can be examined only in terms of comparisons between options. One institution that addresses the need for such comparative effectiveness research, the Patient-Centred Outcomes Research Institute, has as its mandate: 'to improve the quality and relevance of evidence available to help patients, caregivers, clinicians, employers, insurers, and policy makers make informed health decisions.'[119] These are essentially patient-centred questions:[120]

- Given my personal characteristics, conditions and preferences, what should I expect would happen to me?
- What are my options and what are the potential benefits and harms of those options?
- What can I do to improve the outcomes that are most important to me?

This last question is particularly relevant for creating a communication channel with the patient (or, indeed, any healthy person) to examine options in the interlinked practice–research realm and, potentially, to initiate dialogue between various stakeholders. Primary care research and practice should 'borrow from' available approaches, mandates, lessons learned and the overall evidence base to implement and evaluate such patient-centred communication.

CONCLUSION

Patient-centred and integrated care has been the focus of research during the past years. New models to address new challenges are emerging in the literature. The emerging core themes include the need for more compassion and caring in patient interactions as well as the need to have an interdisciplinary approach to the topic. Research into these themes is of particular relevance to primary care.

Patients and healthy persons alike have to be actively involved in the design and evaluation of research, translating the research findings into measurable options and participating in shared and informed decision-making with their providers. Persons should also have a role in implementing research and the actual translation of research findings, allowing them to, ultimately, drive more patient-/person-centred policies.

To that effect, PCR should receive support and attention from governments and policymakers, and other specialties should support the efforts of practitioners in this field through organisations and associations, communities of practice and at all three organisational levels (micro, meso and macro). Also, research in this field should be further supported with strong requirements for impact, dissemination and participatory activities, with the necessary incentives for participants, and particular emphasis on re-training and keeping well-trained and informed practitioners who focus on making research and shared decision-making an integral part of their daily practice. Last, but certainly not least, the efforts to equip practitioners with new skills, new models and interdisciplinary theories of primary care research and practice should allow them not only to participate more actively themselves but also to engage patients or persons in a much more effective and relevant manner.

CHAPTER 10

The contribution of primary care research to improving health services

. . . .

Dee Mangin

INTRODUCTION

It might be assumed that countries that invest more in expensive and highly specialised technological health services secure better outcomes for their citizens. In fact, research has demonstrated that it is investment in the provision of primary care health service delivery that not only improves overall health and longevity of the population but also reduces inequity in distribution of healthcare and health outcomes within a population. Primary care health services research has provided the lens through which this crucial connection has been understood, providing clear guidance on the value of investment in primary care and the importance of the core functions of primary health services as well as the mechanisms by which they may contribute to the effects on health. The intensity, theoretical basis and rigor of this health services research in both providing a comprehensive evidence base for improving health services underpinned by the defining qualities of primary care and investigating the evidence for its effects, effectiveness and cost-effectiveness are unparalleled in any other segment of health service delivery.

THE IMPORTANCE OF PRIMARY CARE TO HEALTH SERVICES

Primary healthcare was first recognised as a distinct domain of health services around 95 years ago, and the first key contribution of primary care research to promoting better healthcare has been to demonstrate the positive impact of primary healthcare on the prevention of illness and of mortality.[121,122] Although there was some research activity in the 1970s–1980s, it was in the 1990s that a significant body of research appeared in the published literature, from a heterogeneous range of settings. A large contribution to both this body of research and to a range of comprehensive analyses and summaries was led by Dr. B Starfield and Dr. L Shi. They published seminal work that analysed, rated and compared different countries on aspects of primary care and correlated these with improved health outcomes.[121, 123,124]

The body of work from primary care health services researchers over this period was able to convincingly demonstrate that the positive effect of primary care service delivery persists across settings and is consistent regardless of which aspect of primary care service delivery is used as a marker (e.g. access, utilisation, enrolment, availability [supply]). From the 1990s, a clear association was demonstrated between primary care physician (PCP) supply and health outcomes, and then, in 2002, a more precise 'dose–response' was articulated.[125-128] A further analysis clarified a year later that, in US studies, it was the supply of family physicians that was related to mortality benefits rather than the other first contact specialist services that were available in the USA.[129]

These studies have provided the compelling evidence base for investment in primary healthcare around the world. Today, the context of most health service delivery in developed countries is primary care: if health services contacts are considered across primary care, specialist visits and hospital admissions, 71% of this healthcare is primary care visits.[130] It should not be surprising, then, that improved outcomes are most closely associated with countries that have the strongest primary care systems.[121]

'Primary care' is the level of a health services system that provides entry into the system for all new needs and problems; provides person-focused (not disease-oriented) care over time; provides care for all but very uncommon or unusual conditions; and coordinates or integrates care, regardless of where the care is delivered and who provides it.

THE KEY DIMENSIONS OF EFFECTIVE PRIMARY CARE

The second key area of contribution of primary care health services research has been to tease out the contribution to effective primary care service delivery of the core attributes of primary healthcare embodied in its definition: first contact care, person-focused care, care over time (continuity, or longitudinal care), comprehensiveness and coordination, again providing evidence to support the evidence base for strengthening these features. The breadth and depth of evidence from primary care research in demonstrating and understanding these effects is similarly unequalled by any other part of the health services. Each of these domains could be reviewed in a chapter of its own – the following is a brief description of each.

Care over time (continuity)

Research beginning decades ago demonstrated the benefits of relational continuity in primary care, in different socioeconomic settings, across a range of outcomes, including uptake of preventive care, improved satisfaction, better adherence, lower hospitalisation and emergency-room use.[131-134] Research on continuity has also shown the core aspects of effective primary care, while able to be separately articulated, are themselves interdependent. The link between relational continuity and increased uptake of primary care services was mediated by patient communication and increased trust as well as increased knowledge of the patient through patient-centred care.[131]

Coordination

'Coordination' is the integration by the primary care practice of all aspects of care when patients are seen elsewhere. Over 20 years ago, the effect of the coordinating role of healthcare was demonstrated. One example of this was research that showed that surgery outcomes were better when patients were referred by their PCP for specialist care than when they self-referred.[135]

First contact care

When the first contact for care within an episode of illness is with primary care, health-care costs are reduced.[136] Other research shows it is first contact with family medicine in primary care rather than other specialist services available in the first contact setting that is linked to mortality benefits, and that, when ongoing care for ambulatory conditions is provided by specialists rather than family physicians, hospitalisation rates are higher independent of variation in patient mix.[129,137]

Person-focused care

Person-focused care is at the heart of primary care; a core value.[138] Research has demonstrated the value of this aspect of primary care across a range of outcomes of relevance to patients: overall quality of life, satisfaction with aspects of service delivery including communication, sensitivity in dealing with problems, trust and treatment adherence.[139,140] Detailed examination has shown again a clear dose–response between a patient-centred approach and patient trust.[141] This work has provided a base for health systems to provide not just efficient and statistically significant care, or disease significant care, or even clinically significant care but, as articulated elegantly by Dr. K Sweeney, care that is of personal significance to the individual.[142]

Comprehensiveness

Patients attending primary care present with a complex array of problems and evidence indicates that the more comprehensive the range of primary care services, the better the results in terms of health outcomes. There is also a higher likelihood of engaging with preventive care across a range of disease contexts and a decreased likelihood of being admitted to hospital.[136,143–145]

These aspects of primary care became a marker for the quality of implementation, and further international comparative studies demonstrated the key for translation of this evidence into practice in service delivery: a strong correlation was demonstrated between supportive government policy and the adequacy of delivery of these key core functions of primary care.[18]

Further analysis of the effects generated from strengthening these core functions of primary care has suggested the mechanisms by which these effects are achieved: greater access to needed services, better quality of care, a greater focus on prevention, early management of health problems, the cumulative effect of the main primary care delivery characteristics and the role of primary care in reducing unnecessary and potentially harmful specialist care.[18] Another body of work demonstrated the value to funders and showed that provision of primary care was associated with lower overall costs to the health system and that weaker primary healthcare had a significant association with higher costs.[146] This is reinforced by condition-specific research demonstrating the same effect: in community-acquired pneumonia (CAP), for example, primary care was associated with lower costs for similar outcomes.[147,148] This was subsequently confirmed in a prospective randomised controlled trial of comprehensive primary care versus hospital-based care for CAP: costs were lower for the same outcomes, and patient satisfaction with primary care was higher.[149]

THE CONTRIBUTION OF PRIMARY CARE TO EQUITY

'Equity', which means using resources cost-effectively in the provision of health services to meet the health needs of populations, is closely related to the principles of distributive justice and also to health equity. Clinical care is not a substitute for the improved social and economic conditions required to close the socio-economic gap in health.[150] Improving health does not necessarily improve inequity – in fact, it can increase it; however, clinical care can and should contribute to reducing health inequity to the extent this is possible.[150] Primary care research has demonstrated how changes in health service delivery can achieve this: in contrast to secondary care, provision of primary care has been shown to promote more equitable distribution of health across a population.[150] It also affects equity in secondary care.[151] The PCP supply has a positive effect on equity in referral patterns to secondary care – for example, increasing referral rates among African Americans relative to those for white Americans for high-cost elective surgical procedures. An addition of one PCP per 1000 people in the USA (tripling current PCP density) would result in a 102% increase in odds of referral-sensitive admissions among blacks, 64% among Hispanics and 36% among whites, relative to marker admissions not sensitive to primary care.[150,151] This was confirmed in implementation research: in the evaluations of healthcare reform centred on strengthening the core aspects of primary care in Spain, Brazil and Thailand, in addition to improved health outcomes, improvements in health equity were also found.

Further work is needed to understand the relative contribution of individual versus population- and political-level strategies to reduce health inequities and of clinical care versus interventions that are more effectively addressed through improved social conditions.[150]

CONTRIBUTION TO QUALITY OF CARE

Measuring and supporting the achievement and maintenance of high-quality primary care remains a challenge. A large body of work has addressed quality in primary care – for instance, in developing conceptual frameworks for comparing models of primary care service delivery,[152] in tools for measuring quality[153] as well as for considering individual- and population-level quality.[154] There is uncertainty about how to best achieve this. Pay-for-performance (P4P) schemes are popular; however, they have met with mixed results and responses and intense debate.[155,156] Further, they are often centred around intermediate surrogates, processes and single diseases rather than more sophisticated measures of system function and service delivery mechanisms. Primary care health services research in the UK has provided rich evidence on the effects of this approach and has been important in demonstrating and beginning to understand the successes and failures within the mixed effect on processes of care and intermediate outcomes.[157–159] There is signposting of the absence of the anticipated positive effect on health outcomes when incentives are clinically based and centred around diseases.[155,160] There is no evidence yet for significant effect on patient-relevant outcomes in primary care: benefit has yet to be demonstrated in premature mortality,[161] in contrast to the use of a P4P approach in secondary care, for which a mortality benefit has been demonstrated, signalling that this disease-focused approach may be more suited to specialist services and not primary care.[162] However, other research shows again the value of the key core functions of primary care: that when the important mechanisms of primary care are functioning well, health outcomes improve with higher quality care – demonstrating, for example, an association between patient-reported ease of access to primary care and reduced hospital admissions across a range of conditions.[163,164]

There is scope for more work in understanding the effects of P4P on the core functions of primary care. There are signals of mixed effects on equity and access and a negative effect on continuity of care, and patient-centredness has been seen, highlighting the potential for opportunity costs along with the lack of anticipated benefit.[160] There is little evidence on the effect of P4P on coordination and comprehensiveness, although, for the latter, there is some evidence of a decline in attention when conditions are not incentivised.[165]

IMPLEMENTATION OF PRIMARY CARE

Beyond these correlations, primary care research has also been able to demonstrate the effect of countries implementing this evidence-based approach in primary healthcare services from the 1980s onwards: for example, Spain strengthened primary care in the mid-1980s by reorganising services to better align with the core mechanisms by which primary healthcare achieves improved outcomes, establishing a national programme of primary care centres. The subsequent impact of this reform was evaluated a decade later using mortality from major causes of death. This research found a clear association between the process of reform of primary care and the decrease in general mortality in the low socio-economic areas in which the reforms were implemented. Death rates associated with stroke and hypertension fell most in those zones in which reform was first implemented (1984–1989) compared with in those where it was implemented later (1989–1991).[166] Similar effects, as well as increased patient satisfaction, were found in research into the effect of investment in primary care service delivery in both Brazil and Thailand, where the balance of health services was deliberately shifted away from specialised hospital-based service to primary care.[101,167–172] Portugal has seen perhaps the most striking gains in health outcomes by implementing health services centred on the core primary care attributes.[101]

CONCLUSION

Good healthcare requires the integration of three things: the recognition of the patient's problems by a practitioner with the empathy to understand their story, consideration of the best that medical science has to offer, and a system of service delivery most likely to translate this into care that will improve or maintain the life of that individual. Of these three aspects, two are constantly changing: patient problems and medical science. Aside from contributing accurate data on the effectiveness and safety of treatments, primary care research has played, and will continue to play, a central role in articulating the key aspects of healthcare service delivery that improve health and health equity. As the pattern of illness has changed in ageing populations to one of multi-morbidity, primary care systems and primary care research must rise to the challenge of demonstrating the aspects of service delivery that make it fit for purpose in this changing context. This is starting to happen, with comprehensive descriptions of the change in patterns of morbidity and the implications for care in different contexts, although not quickly enough.[173–176]

The 2008 World Health Organization (WHO) report *Primary Health Care: Now More than Ever* comprehensively articulates the importance of strong and effective primary care for health.[101] The fact that it is able to make this argument stands on the collective contribution of primary care research. The challenge for policymakers and funders is to support the generation, testing and integration of primary healthcare research in evidence-based policies and funding models. Funding models designed not just for contacts and conditions, but that recognise the importance of effective primary care delivery and the important primary care characteristics that underpin its effectiveness. The WHO report was a call to action for primary care service delivery; the same applies to the value of primary care research, now more than ever.

CHAPTER 11

Financing, leadership, governance and primary care health systems research

....

Luisa Pettigrew[*]

INTRODUCTION

The World Health Organization (WHO) outlines six 'building blocks' that are needed to achieve the overall goals – (1) improving health, (2) being responsive, (3) providing social and financial risk protection, (4) improving efficiency, (5) financing, and (6) leadership/governance – of a health system[177] (Figure 11.1).

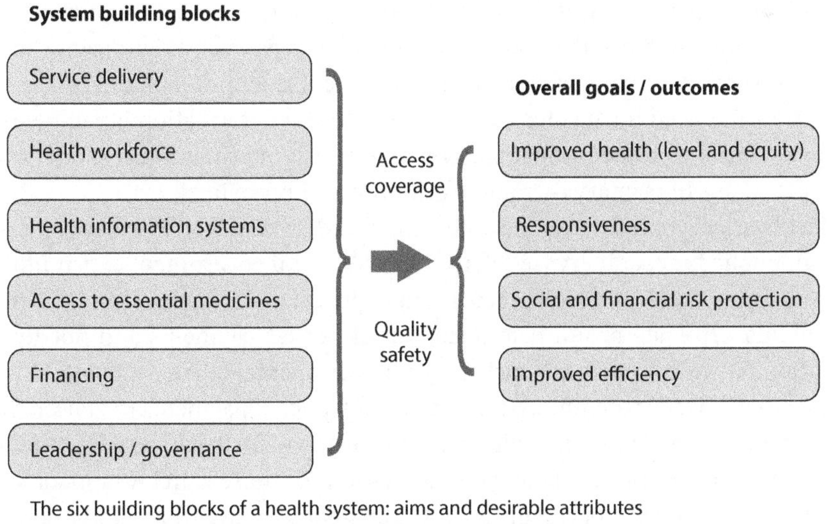

System building blocks

Service delivery

Health workforce

Health information systems

Access to essential medicines

Financing

Leadership / governance

Access coverage

Quality safety

Overall goals / outcomes

Improved health (level and equity)

Responsiveness

Social and financial risk protection

Improved efficiency

The six building blocks of a health system: aims and desirable attributes

FIGURE 11.1 The WHO Health Systems Framework[177]

* Luisa Pettigrew is funded by an NIHR In-Practice Fellowship. The views expressed are those of the author and not necessarily those of the NHS, the NIHR or Department of Health.

With primary care research in mind, this chapter focuses on the last two building blocks of *financing* and *leadership/governance*. Effective financing mechanisms, leadership and governance are needed to invest in and deliver good-quality primary care research. Conversely, good-quality primary care research is necessary to inform evidence-based policymaking regarding financing mechanisms, leadership and governance structure in order to fully realise the potential of primary care within any health system. Moreover, an interrelationship clearly exists between good leadership, governance and effectively financed health systems.

This chapter therefore aims to offer an overview of the role of primary care research in relation to the financing and leadership/governance building blocks in the WHO framework. It does so by offering an outline of definitions and measures of these building blocks and providing examples from a global and a country-level perspective of the roles and interrelationship of the building blocks with regards to primary care and primary care research.

DEFINITIONS AND MEASURES

'Health system financing' in essence refers to how funds are collected, pooled and then spent to run a health system,[177] Numerous measures of how health systems are financed exist.[178] For example, total health expenditure (THE), as a percentage of gross domestic product (GDP), or per capita expenditure on health is often used to compare healthcare expenditure across countries. Ideally, the percentage of THE or per capita expenditure on primary care should also be routinely measured. However, although there is important research into this across a number of higher income countries,[121,179] the ability to accurately measure primary care expenditure in many countries worldwide is still limited due to the poor availability of data as well as significant challenges in defining and identifying what primary care does / does not include. This is an area with a pressing need for further research, as with this information it will be possible to provide more accurate comparisons on investment in primary care, better evaluate the effectiveness of primary care and work towards improving it.

Healthcare expenditure can also be considered in terms of whether it is paid for through public funds, otherwise referred to as 'general government expenditure' (i.e. taxation and compulsory/social security insurance), or through private expenditure (i.e. voluntary/private health insurance, out of pocket payments and not-for-profit institutions serving households such as non-governmental organisations).[178] Evidence suggests that private expenditure through out-of-pocket payments (e.g. user charges, co-payments) is the least equitable mechanism to pay for healthcare, as it results in the greatest financial burden falling on the sick and/or those with lower incomes.[180–182] Moreover, out-of-pocket payments do not consistently reduce what may be considered the 'unnecessary' use of health services, but, rather, often delay the presentation of conditions that would have been less costly had they been addressed sooner, resulting in overall health system inefficiencies.[180–182] Therefore, measures such as 'catastrophic out-of-pocket expenditure', defined as when a household's financial contribution to the health system exceeds 40% of income remaining after subsistence needs have been met, are important indicators of how well, or not, a health system is providing financial risk protection.[183]

In terms of 'leadership' and 'governance', WHO defines these as, 'ensuring that strategic policy frameworks exist and are combined with effective oversight, coalition-building, regulation, attention to system design and accountability'.[177] Indicators of leadership and governance can be rules or outcomes based. For example, whether appropriate policies, strategies and approaches to support good leadership and governance exist can be used as indicators. Alternatively, whether the rules and procedures are effectively applied and whether they have resulted in the desired outcomes can be measured. Research can be used to answer important questions such as: Are there policies on primary care and primary care research that explicitly define the vision for the future? Do they outline how objectives will be achieved? Who will be responsible for this and who are they accountable to? How will success be measured? How will failures be addressed?

Financing decisions and the associated leadership and governance structures are relevant across primary care clinical, organisational, academic and policy domains, at local, regional, national and international levels. The following subsections offer global and country-level perspectives on the role of financing, leadership and governance decisions on primary care and primary care research, and vice versa.

A GLOBAL PERSPECTIVE

One of the biggest challenges primary care has faced and continues to struggle with is defining itself. How different stakeholders, whether providers, the public, policymakers or funders, interpret the term 'primary care' can vary. This has historically had significant implications in relation to financing, leadership and governance decisions, and it is something that primary care research has helped address and needs to continue to do so.

The *Declaration of Alma-Ata* advocated for the delivery of comprehensive, community-based, people-centred care through the delivery of primary healthcare in 1978.[184] However, over the years that followed, the appeal of funding specific conditions with quicker and easier to measure results led many countries to shift their focus to the support of vertically (i.e. disease/condition specific) oriented programmes, often referred to as 'selective primary care'. Likewise, while the Millennium Development Goals catalysed laudable improvements in health in many countries, they have also had well-recognised shortcomings due to their emphasis on vertical programmes. Research evidence now suggests that the dominance of vertical programme approaches in many settings has contributed to fragmented and weak health systems. Meanwhile, leading primary care research by Barbara Starfield and others has helped to both define the dimensions of primary care that make it successful and quantify its benefits.[179,180,185,186] As a result, in recent years, the global discourse has started to shift back to the need to invest in health system strengthening and comprehensive primary care.[101,187]

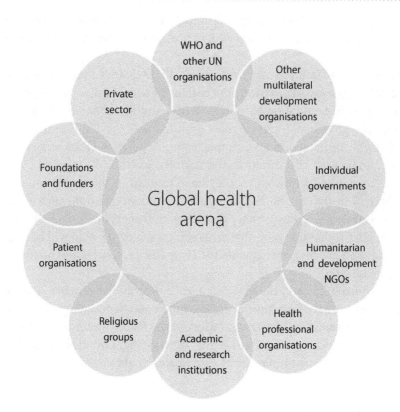

FIGURE 11.2 Actors in the global health arena

The United Nations, through organisations such as the World Bank and WHO, has played a growing role in global health governance since these organisations were established after World War II. In the last few decades, however, the number of actors in the global health arena has expanded rapidly, with philanthropic and other non-governmental organisations, including the private sector, playing a much greater role (Figure 11.2).

Each actor has its own agenda and responds to different stakeholders with different interests. This both presents opportunities and challenges in terms of creating cohesive leadership and governance structures that will result in greater investment in primary care research in order to strengthen primary care. Significant work is still needed for there to be a consistent investment into primary care research across high-, middle- and low-income countries alike and for those responsible for global health governance to act appropriately in response to the evidence. Promises regarding investing in health system strengthening and in primary care should be approached with caution, and what is meant by these terms should be questioned.[188] Sparse reference to investment in primary care research in *The World Health Report 2013: Research for Universal Health Coverage*[189] and limited reference to indicators that will enable the measurement of comprehensive primary care in drafts of the Sustainable Development

Goals[190] are a reflection of the significant challenges that persist in the field of global health development.

A COUNTRY-LEVEL PERSPECTIVE

At country level, how funding flows to primary care and primary care research will determine what is delivered, by who, where, when and how. Making decisions on funding allocation is complex, involves many stakeholders and will always be political in nature. This reinforces why good leadership and governance, informed by solid evidence, based on the needs of local populations, are essential. Agreeing on how to distribute public funds in the most effective, efficient and equitable way is hugely challenging. For example, inadequate risk adjustment formulae that do not fairly take into consideration the extra resources associated with caring for sicker, older or disadvantaged populations when allocating funds can result in the inequitable distribution of resources and care.

There is broad agreement that 'primary care' (defined as person-centred, comprehensive, integrated and continuous care, with a regular point of entry into the health system, that allows a relationship of trust between people and their healthcare providers[101]), is an essential, cost-effective and equitable means to help achieve 'universal health coverage' (defined as 'for all people to be able use the health services they need, of sufficient quality to be effective, while also ensuring that the use of these services does not expose the user to financial hardship'[191]). Therefore, with the evidence regarding the impact of out-of-pocket payments described earlier in mind, the use of out-of-pocket payment in primary care is likely to be detrimental to the objective of achieving universal health coverage and emphasises the importance of both undertaking research into the impact of how primary care is financed and conveying this to funders, policymakers as well as the public and providers.

How providers are paid is important too. Although remuneration is not the only mechanism that can influence the behaviour of providers, there is a body of research studying how being paid by a salary, fee for service, capitation or pay-for-performance results in different behaviour in family doctors and can modify their clinical practice as well as encourage or disincentivise collaboration with other parts of the health system.[192,193] Poorly aligned and perverse incentives for primary care providers, under-the-table payments and outright corruption are a reflection of poor financing systems and weak governance and leadership. Primary care–based research is needed to highlight these challenges and identify potential solutions within the relevant country context.

There is also growing evidence on the role of financial incentives to change patients' behaviour – for example, payments to incentivise health-seeking behaviour, such as antenatal care, or financial incentives to encourage patients to access primary care before secondary care.[110,183] However, more primary care–based research across varying contexts is needed to truly understand whether such policies are transferable to different economic, political and cultural settings and what role they can play.

Guidelines based on cost-effectiveness analyses of clinical interventions and drugs are playing an increasing role in many countries in order to inform decisions regarding what services and drugs should be funded. These evaluations are based on research evidence; however, the basis of this research is increasingly challenged due both to links with the pharmaceutical industry and because it is often undertaken on very specific populations (e.g. below a certain age, with only one condition) and therefore does not reflect the reality of populations seen in primary care. For instance, there is inadequate primary care research into patients with complex multi-morbidity despite this becoming increasingly common in many settings.[194] This again highlights the pressing need for transparent primary care–based research to inform funding policy decisions, as well as the development of clinical guidance.

It is important to highlight that the responsibility for good leadership and governance falls not only in the domain of policymakers; it is also the responsibility of all the other stakeholders, including clinicians and the public. Clinical governance and clinical leadership are increasingly recognised as an important part of clinical training and ongoing professional development.[195,196] Clinicians who bridge the fields of academia, management and policymaking are fundamental to the improvement of health systems. The contribution of patients, their families and the public at large is also being increasingly recognised as a vital part of the governance of any health system. However, while there is growing work in this area, many questions remain unanswered about how to best enable and meaningfully utilise public engagement to improve primary care in different settings.[197,198]

CONCLUSION

There are clear links between health system spending, leadership and governance. Carefully considered financing systems, good leadership and robust governance structures are needed to support high-quality primary care service delivery and primary care research. Likewise, primary care–based research is essential for developing relevant and evidence-based policymaking regarding health systems financing, leadership and governance at local, national and international levels.

The WHO *World Health Report 2008* highlighted[101] 'it is remarkable that an industry that currently mobilizes 8.6% of the world's GDP invests so little in research on two of its most effective and cost-effective strategies: primary care and the public policies that underpin and complement it … No other I$5 trillion economic sector would be happy with so little investment in research related to its core agenda: the reduction of health inequalities; the organization of people-centred care; and the development of better, more effective public policies'.

While there is indication that interest in investing in primary care research is growing, in order to realise the full potential of primary care and improve the financing, leadership and governance building blocks of any health system, much greater efforts are needed to invest in primary care and primary care research on a global scale.

CHAPTER 12

The contribution of primary care research to education, training and development of the primary healthcare workforce

· ·

Wim Peersman and Jan De Maeseneer

INTRODUCTION: HUMAN RESOURCES AND EDUCATIONAL RESEARCH

Human resources are key in the development of policies to strengthen primary health-care (PHC) systems worldwide. In their 2009 editorial 'Renewed focus on primary health care (PHC)' in *Education for Health*, Glasser and Pathman emphasise the need for research on PHC education.[199]

Educational research on human resources has to take into account the framework offered by the report 'Health professionals for a new century: transforming education to strengthen health systems in an interdependent world'.[200] In the previous century, research mainly focused on assessment of problem-based learning and disciplinarily integrated curricula. Didactical innovations were evaluated, including the use of standardised patients to assess a student's clinical practice, the impact of earlier student exposure to patients and the expansion of training sites from hospitals to communities. The majority of this research was conducted in high-income countries, and only a few studies documented developments in low- and middle-income countries (LMICs).

The Lancet Commission indicates that, in the twenty-first century, a third generation of reforms is needed that should be system based to improve the performance of health systems by adapting core professional competencies to specific contexts, while drawing on global knowledge.[200] The realisation of this vision will require reforms with two important outcomes: transformative learning and interdependence in education. 'Transformative learning' is about developing leadership attributes with the intention to produce change agents. 'Interdependence' is a key element in a systems approach and involves three fundamental shifts: from isolated educational programmes to programmes harmonised with health systems; from stand-alone institutions to networks; and from inward-looking institutional preoccupations to harnessing global flows of educational content, teaching resources and innovations.[200]

The challenge nowadays is to start using the framework of this third generation of reforms to formulate new research questions that will also require new methodological approaches, such as mixed methods and participatory action research. PHC represents an important field of research in order to test the third-generation reforms: experiences such as community-based education and service (COBES) create opportunities to evaluate how educational innovation has made undergraduate and postgraduate medical training more relevant to the needs of PHC. The Network: Towards Unity For Health has documented the evaluation of many of these community-based educational initiatives.[201] The Training for Health Equity Network[202] also uses a systems perspective,

---

BOX 12.1 Recommendations to transform and scale up health professionals' education and training (selection)[203]

- Health professionals' education and training institutions should consider designing and implementing continuous development programmes for faculty and teaching staff relevant to the evolving health-care needs of their communities.
- Health professionals' education and training institutions should consider innovative expansion of faculty, through the recruitment of community-based clinicians and health workers as educators.
- Health professionals' education and training institutions should consider adapting curricula to the evolving health-care needs of their communities.
- Health professionals' education and training institutions should use simulation methods (high fidelity methods in settings with appropriate resources and lower fidelity methods in resource limited settings) of contextually appropriate fidelity levels in the education of health professionals.
- Health professionals' education and training institutions should consider using targeted admissions policies to increase the socio-economic, ethnic and geographical diversity of students.
- Health professionals' education and training institutions should consider implementing inter-professional education (IPE) in both undergraduate and postgraduate programmes.
- National governments should introduce accreditation of health professionals' education where it does not exist and strengthen it where it does exist.
- Health professionals' education and training institutions should consider implementing continuous professional development and in-service training of health professionals relevant to the evolving health-care needs of their communities.

looking at ways to increase social accountability and reorient educational programmes towards the needs of society.

The *Transforming and Scaling Up Health Professionals' Education and Training* guidelines from WHO[203] summarise the current evidence in relation to the evaluation of health professional education in recommendations across five domains: education and training institutions, accreditation and regulation, financing and sustainability, monitoring and evaluating, and governance and planning (Box 12.1).

In this chapter we illustrate, using the example of the Human Resources for African Primary Health Care (HURAPRIM) project, how primary care research can help tackle human resource issues from a systems perspective, focusing on brain drain, problems with access, need for optimisation of service delivery, importance of task-shifting and competency sharing. The chapter ends with a reflection on social accountability and dissemination, extremely relevant for this type of research, and finally, formulates a critical reflection on 'societal impact'.

ADDRESSING THE HUMAN RESOURCES CRISIS: THE HURAPRIM ACTION-RESEARCH PROJECT

In 2011, the HURAPRIM project started looking at the challenge of recruitment, training and retention of human resources for African PHC. In this section, we describe the aims of the HURAPRIM project, explore the research questions and describe the different interventions as an illustration of how primary care research can contribute to the development of an appropriate health workforce for the health system.

Aims of the HURAPRIM project

Several reports have documented the huge deficit of human resources for health (HRH) in Africa.[204,205] The causes are multiple and relate to a combination of underproduction, internal maldistribution, inappropriate task allocation, working conditions and brain drain. The main objective of the HURAPRIM project was to analyse the actual situation of HRH in Africa and to understand the complexity of the causes for the actual shortages in PHC. Based on these results, the project developed innovative interventions, strategies and policies to address the HRH crisis in sub-Saharan Africa and evaluated those interventions, strategies and policies. Five African countries were involved (Mali, Sudan, Uganda, Botswana and South Africa), representing Africa's broad diversity.

Research methods used for the HURAPRIM project

First, the project assessed the scope of the deficit in HRH in Africa and identified and analysed its main causes, with special emphasis on PHC in rural areas and underserved urban areas. The research tasks for this objective consisted of four components:

1. A literature review (including grey literature) on the availability of health workers in the participating African countries, compared with what would be needed to provide access to healthcare for the relevant populations.[205]

2. Participatory research with stakeholders in selected districts of the included African countries to determine what human resources were currently available in the health sector, what gaps existed in service provision, what the reasons were for the deficit in human resources, which interventions had already been tried and ideas for new interventions.[206]

3. A confidential enquiry into maternal and child deaths in Mali and Uganda. This approach consisted of an independent review of a series of deaths that explicitly avoided attributing blame to individuals but attempted to identify modifiable system failures. The cases were summarised and presented to a panel of local health workers (nurses, general practitioners and hospital specialists) and community representatives, with the aim of prioritising how human resources for health could best be used to reduce maternal and child mortality.

4. Semi-structured interviews with migrant health workers in partner countries that receive migrant health workers (UK, Belgium and Austria in Europe, and South Africa and Botswana in Africa) to find out their reasons for migration (push and pull factors), what might motivate them to return to their country of origin to work in the health sector and to get their perspective on reasons for the lack of health workers in Africa.

Based on the results of this first phase, the following interventions were developed, implemented, monitored and evaluated in the participating African countries.

Primary healthcare re-engineering, including primary healthcare outreach teams, as a human resources strategy in South Africa

In South Africa, the Chiawelo Community Practice developed a community-oriented primary care model, coordinated by a family physician, that was based on PHC outreach teams consisting of community health workers led by professional nurses. This offered an opportunity to explore the development of integrated PHC teamwork in South Africa. To translate the research into action, the participatory action research method was used.[206] This method included qualitative and quantitative approaches but was, above all, participative. The key advantage of using an action research method was that it drew attention to how an intervention unfolds and how the actions of an intervention can mutually benefit a community of practitioners.

Confidential enquiry in Uganda and Mali as action research aimed at improving quality of primary healthcare delivery

The aim of this intervention was to refine the confidential enquiry process into a tool that could be scaled up and used both to improve quality of human resources and to prioritise and advocate for more human resources in areas of greatest need. The process included a strong element of dissemination of results at all levels from the community to health workers to politicians. The primary outcome measure was the number of child (under 5 years) deaths in the selected sub-counties in year 2 compared with in year 1. From this, and official statistics on populations of the sub-counties, and estimated birth rates, it was also possible to estimate the under-5 mortality rate. Secondary outcome measures included implementation of recommendations to improve quality. In addition, focus groups discussions with participants and in-depth interviews with key stakeholders were conducted on how they evaluated the intervention.

Strengthening of the supportive supervisory capacity of primary care teams via the district health management team and mid-level health managers in Botswana

A cooperative inquiry group (CIG) was used to build the supportive supervision practice of the district health management teams (DHMTs) and cluster heads. The use of the CIG method falls within the participatory action research paradigm.[207] The CIG was composed of the DHMT and mid-level health managers in the district (cluster heads). The aim of the intervention was to explore whether strengthening the supportive supervisory practice of the DHMT and mid-level health managers could improve retention of PHC workers. A survey was also used to evaluate changes in healthcare workers' motivation to remain in PHC and in their perceptions of organisational culture and to compare this with a non-intervention district.[208]

Promoting cooperation between Western schooled and traditional primary healthcare workers in Mali

The main objective was to reduce maternal and neonatal mortality, and to promote low-risk motherhood, by an organised and evaluated collaboration between traditional and modern health systems through participatory action research. More specifically, traditional birth attendants were involved in the management of obstetric emergencies and in the promotion of low-risk motherhood. Another objective was to define and set up a sustainable and participatory village-level data collection and reporting process on maternal and neonatal health by strengthening the local health information system.

Ethical considerations

During all the research activities, the major ethical challenges related to brain drain and the human resource crisis in African PHC were identified to design an ethical framework that could be used to stimulate the ethical debate on human resources for health.

SOCIAL ACCOUNTABILITY AND DISSEMINATION

Scientific work on human resources for African PHC is not a 'neutral' exercise and confronts researchers with the societal need to provide 'scientific evidence' in the midst of important debates. In 2012, there was a debate in the Ugandan parliament, with many MPs initially insisting they would not pass the national budget if the government did not reverse its plan to reduce health expenditure. However, according to the 2012/2013 national budget framework paper,[209] the health ministry budget was going to be reduced substantially.

Primary care researchers of HURAPRIM, in cooperation with the Department of

Family Medicine of Mbarara University of Science and Technology, decided to provide a four-page informative document entitled 'Why Uganda needs to increase its health budget: a briefing for MPs',[209] summarising the evidence and documenting the actual challenges – for example, the death of too many mothers and children in Uganda. After the debate, the government announced that it would double the monthly pay for doctors in level IV health centres and would spend extra money to recruit 6172 health workers.

Apart from these 'contextual opportunities' to disseminate findings, an active strategy using a variety of media is necessary. For example, in May 2015, a short document entitled 'Supporting family practice in Africa', based on the HURAPRIM project, was published by the European Commission (Box 12.2).[210]

BOX 12.2 'Supporting family practice in Africa'[210]

What good is an empty clinic? The brain drain that is depleting healthcare services in many parts of Africa is leaving entire communities stranded. An EU-funded project is looking into ways to mobilise more human resources for primary healthcare across the continent.

The HURAPRIM project focuses on primary healthcare in Africa. It strives to shed new light on the reasons why the human resources required to run these services are hard to recruit and retain and aims to identify strategies that could help to turn the situation around.

Due to end in May 2015, the HURAPRIM project – implemented jointly by partner organisations in Austria, Belgium, Botswana, Mali, Sudan, South Africa, Uganda and the United Kingdom – has analysed the motivations of health workers who have decided to migrate and the impact of these departures on public health. It has also taken steps to raise awareness of the importance of primary healthcare services, highlighted promising strategies to boost human resources in frontline services and issued recommendations for policy-makers.

Treating the brain drain

While many healthcare workers leave to work in other continents, says project coordinator Jan De Maeseneer of Ghent University, there is also a brain drain phenomenon within Africa. Human resources are moving from rural areas to the cities, from primary care to specialty care, from the public service to private services, and from general healthcare to programmes focusing on specific diseases such as HIV/AIDS, he explains.

'There are economic and political elements that determine the fact that people migrate: difficult work conditions, low salaries, and very high workloads,' De Maeseneer notes. Economic conditions are of course an important factor, he explains, but many people emigrate for other reasons – to specialise in a particular field, for example, to escape political instability or insecurity, or to join family members who are already living abroad.

These are understandable personal decisions, often taken in very difficult circumstances, says De Maeseneer. Strategies to counter the phenomenon need to focus on structural solutions that boost health workers' options at home.

Addressing the problem is not simply a matter of money, De Maeseneer explains, although of course adequate financial resources are needed. Training health workers in their own country would, for example, already solve part of the problem. While a number of African countries have excellent facilities in place to train prospective health workers, others do not – and persons who have already left for their studies often decide to remain abroad.

Specific strategies to support family practice in underserved areas would be another option. Medical graduates willing to work in remote rural locations could receive additional training and support over the internet, for example, enabling them to build up the required skills and autonomy.

A healthcare emergency

HURAPRIM looked into the causes of brain drain, but it also examined the consequences – for example by means of 'virtual autopsies' of children deceased under the age of five. The researchers interviewed the families and health workers involved in a number of cases and concluded that most of these tragedies could have been prevented. Where primary healthcare is unavailable or underskilled, lives are lost.

Armed with this information, HURAPRIM was able to document this fact in its interaction with policy-makers. 'In the places where we did this kind of intervention, deaths decreased in the following years,' De Maeseneer reports.

Be fair

HURAPRIM is preparing a list of recommendations for policy-makers both in Africa and abroad. Indeed, countries recruiting health workers from less affluent countries also bear part of the responsibility, says De Maeseneer.

This observation shapes one of HURAPRIM's key messages. 'The international community should agree that if you integrate a doctor or a nurse that was trained in a developing country in your health system in the West, you should reimburse the full cost of training that person to the country of origin,' De Maeseneer explains.

The amount of this refund should correspond to the much higher cost of training such a person in the recruiting country, he adds. This approach would enable countries of origin to train several people for every person that has left. 'This is the least we should do if we take advantage of the training people received elsewhere,' De Maeseneer concludes.

CONCLUSION

We have used the experience of the HURAPRIM project to illustrate the need for a comprehensive research approach when it comes to the important human resource challenges in African PHC. This African experience can be broadened to an international context and educational primary care research can be one of the strategies to address human resource problems. Action research and the use of mixed methods are useful approaches to addressing the reforms outlined in the report of The Lancet Commission.[200] Integration of a systems perspective in the research will also avoid the risk of jumping to simple (but incomplete) one-dimensional conclusions. Involving the broader societal context is essential. Moreover, it is important that researchers use appropriate ways to disseminate the findings of the research to increase the social accountability of scientific work and contribute to 'societal impact'.[211,212]

ACKNOWLEDGEMENTS

This work was conducted as part of the HURAPRIM project, an international collaborative research programme funded by the EUFP7 Africa-Call-2010 under grant agreement no. 265727: http://www.huraprim-project.eu.

SECTION II REFERENCES

1. GBD 2013 Mortality and Causes of Death Collaborators. Global, regional, and national age-sex specific all-cause and cause-specific mortality for 240 causes of death, 1990–2013: a systematic analysis for the Global Burden of Disease Study 2013. *Lancet* 2015; **385**(9963): 117–71.

2. Mant D. Preventive medicine. In: Warrell DA, Cox TM, Firth JD, editors. *Oxford Textbook of Medicine*. Vol. 1. 4th ed. Oxford: Oxford University Press, 2010. pp. 58–63 (online access to the *Oxford Textbook of Medicine* in low- and middle-income countries is available through the World Health Organization-led Health Inter-Network Access to Research Initiative (HINARI)).

3. Imperial Cancer Research Fund General Practice Research Group. Effectiveness of a nicotine patch in helping people stop smoking: results of a randomised trial in general practice. *BMJ* 1993; **306**(6888): 1304–8.

4. Family Heart Study Group. Randomised controlled trial evaluating cardiovascular screening and intervention in general practice: principal results of British family heart study. *BMJ* 1994; **308**(6924): 313–20.

5. Hartmann-Boyce J, Stead LF, Cahill K et al. Efficacy of interventions to combat tobacco addiction: Cochrane update of 2012 reviews. *Addiction* 2013; **108**(10): 1711–21.

6. Mant D. Health checks and screening: what works in general practice? *British Journal of General Practice* 2014; **64**(627): 493–4.

7. Johnson S. *The Ghost Map: The Story of London's Most Terrifying Epidemic – and How It Changed Science, Cities, and the Modern World*. London: Penguin, 2006.

8. Thompson MJ, Ninis N, Perera R et al. Clinical recognition of meningococcal disease in children and adolescents. *Lancet* 2006; **367**(9508): 397–403.

9. Little P, Stuart B, Moore M et al.; GRACE consortium. Amoxicillin for acute lower-respiratory-tract infection in primary care when pneumonia is not suspected: a 12-country, randomised, placebo-controlled trial. *Lancet Infectious Diseases* 2013; **13**(2): 123–9.

10. Williamson I, Vennik J, Harnden A et al. Effect of nasal balloon autoinflation in children with otitis media with effusion in primary care: an open randomised controlled trial. *Canadian Medical Association Journal* 2015; **187**(13): 961–9.

11. Medical Research Council Working Party. MRC trial of treatment of mild hypertension: principal results. *British Medical Journal (Clinical Research Edition)* 1985; **291**(6488): 97–104.

12. Griffin S. Diabetes care in general practice: meta-analysis of randomised control trials. *BMJ* 1998; **317**(7155): 390–6.

13. Drummond N, Abdalla M, Buckingham JK et al.; Grampian Asthma Study of Integrated Care (GRASSIC) Investigators. Integrated care for asthma: a clinical, social, and economic evaluation. *BMJ* 1994; **308**(6928): 559–64.

14. Horne R, Mailey E, Frost S et al. Shared care: a qualitative study of GPs' and hospital doctors' views on prescribing specialist medicine. *British Journal of General Practice* 2001; **51**(464): 181–93.

15. Rowe AK, de Savigny D, Lanata CF et al. How can we achieve and maintain high-quality performance of health workers in low-resource settings? *Lancet* 2005; **366**(9490): 1026–35.

16. Blacklock C, Gonçalves Bradley D, Mickan S et al. Impact of contextual factors on the effect of interventions to improve health worker performance in sub-Saharan Africa: review of randomised clinical trials. *PLoS ONE* 2016; **11**(1): e0145206.

17. Allen T, Mason T, Whittaker W. Impacts of pay for performance on the quality of primary care. *Risk Management and Healthcare Policy* 2014; **7**: 113–20.

18. Sackett DL. How to read clinical journals: I. why to read them and how to start reading them critically. *Can Med Assoc J* 1981; Mar 1; **124**(5): 555–8.

19. Guyatt GH. Evidence-based medicine. *American College of Physicians Journal Club* 1991; **114**: A16.
20. Guyatt GH, Rennie D. Users' guides to the medical literature. *JAMA* 1993; **270**(17): 2096–7.
21. Starr M, Chalmers I, Clarke M et al. The origins, evolution, and future of *The Cochrane Database of Systematic Reviews*. *International Journal of Technology Assessment in Health Care* 2009; **25** (Suppl. 1): 182–95.
22. Smith R, Rennie D. Evidence-based medicine – an oral history. *JAMA* 2014; **311**(4): 365–7.
23. AGREE Collaboration. Development and validation of an international appraisal instrument for assessing the quality of clinical practice guidelines: the AGREE project. *Quality and Safety in Health Care* **15**(1): 17–22 2003; **12**(1): 18–23.
24. McElduff P, Lyratzopoulos G, Edwards R et al. Will changes in primary care improve health outcomes? Modelling the impact of financial incentives introduced to improve quality of care in the UK. *Quality and Safety in Health Care* 2004; **13**(3): 191–7.
25. Goodyear-Smith F. Practising alchemy: the transmutation of evidence into best health care. *Family Practice* 2011; **28**(2): 123–7.
26. Sackett DL, Rosenberg WM, Gray JA et al. Evidence based medicine: what it is and what it isn't. *BMJ* 1996; **312**(7023): 71–2.
27. Edwards N, Barker PM. The importance of context in implementation research. *Journal of Acquired Immune Deficiency Syndromes* 2014; **67** (Suppl. 2): S157–62.
28. Jagosh J, Macaulay AC, Pluye P et al. Uncovering the benefits of participatory research: implications of a realist review for health research and practice. *Milbank Quarterly* 2012; **90**(2): 311–46.
29. Chambers DA, Glasgow RE, Stange KC. The dynamic sustainability framework: addressing the paradox of sustainment amid ongoing change. *Implementation Science* 2013; **8**: 117.
30. Greenhalgh T, Robert G, Macfarlane F et al. Diffusion of innovations in service organizations: systematic review and recommendations. *Milbank Quarterly* 2004; **82**(4): 581–629.
31. Peters DH, Tran NT, Adam T. *Implementation Research in Health: A Practical Guide*. Geneva: World Health Organization (WHO), 2013. Available at: http://apps.who.int/iris/bitstream/10665/91758/1/9789241506212_eng.pdf?ua=1 (accessed 27 November 2015).
32. Brennan TA, Leape LL, Laird NM et al. Incidence of adverse events and negligence in hospitalized patients: results of the Harvard Medical Practice Study I. *New England Journal of Medicine* 1991; **324**(6): 370–6.
33. Kohn LT, Corrigan JM, Donaldson MS, editors; Committee on Quality of Health Care in America, Institute of Medicine, authors. *To Err Is Human: Building a Safer Health System*. Washington DC: National Academies Press, 2000.
34. Vincent C, Neale G, Woloshynowych M. Adverse events in British hospitals: preliminary retrospective record review. *BMJ* 2001; **322**(7285): 517–19.
35. Makeham MA, Kidd MR, Saltman DC et al. The Threats to Australian Patient Safety (TAPS) study: incidence of reported errors in general practice. *Medical Journal of Australia* 2006; **185**(2): 95–8.
36. Tsang C, Majeed A, Banarsee R et al. Recording of adverse events in English general practice: analysis of data from electronic patient records. *Informatics in Primary Care* 2010; **18**(2): 117–24.
37. Wetzels R, Wolters R, van Weel C et al. Harm caused by adverse events in primary care: a clinical observational study. *Journal of Evaluation in Clinical Practice* 2009; **15**(2): 323–7.
38. National Health Service (NHS) Scotland. Scottish Patient Safety Programme [homepage]. Available at: http://www.scottishpatientsafetyprogramme.scot.nhs.uk/programme (accessed 12 May 2015).

39. Shojania KG, Thomas EJ. Trends in adverse events over time: why are we not improving? *BMJ Quality & Safety* 2013; **22**: 273–7.

40. May CR, Finch TL, Cornford J et al. Integrating telecare for chronic disease management in the community: what needs to be done? *BMC Health Services Research* 2011; **11**: 131.

41. Schierhout G, Hains J, Si D et al. Evaluating the effectiveness of a multifaceted, multilevel continuous quality improvement programme in primary health care: developing a realist theory of change. *Implementation Science* 2013; **8**: 119.

42. US Department of Health and Human Services. *Code of Federal Regulations: Title 45 Public Welfare; Department of Health and Human Services – Part 46 Protection of Human Subjects.* 45 CRF 46. Washington DC: US Department of Health and Human Services, 2009. Available at: http://www.hhs.gov/ohrp/policy/ohrpregulations.pdf. Last accessed 12 May 2015.

43. Rosser W, Dovey S, Bordman R et al. Medical errors in primary care: results of an international study of family practice. *Canadian Family Physician* 2005; **51**: 386–7.

44. de Wet C, Bowie P. The preliminary development and testing of a global trigger tool to detect error and patient harm in primary-care records. *Postgraduate Medical Journal* 2009; **85**(1002): 176–80.

45. Woods DM, Thomas EJ, Holl JL et al. Ambulatory care adverse events and preventable adverse events leading to a hospital admission. *Quality and Safety in Health Care* 2007; **16**(2): 127–31.

46. Rubin G, George A, Chinn DJ et al. Errors in general practice: development of an error classification and pilot study of a method for detecting errors. *Quality and Safety in Health Care* 2003; **12**(6): 443–7.

47. Garfield S, Barber N, Walley P et al. Quality of medication use in primary care – mapping the problem, working to a solution: a systematic review of the literature. *BMC Medicine* 2009; **7**: 50.

48. Tache SV, Sonnichsen A, Ashcroft DM. Prevalence of adverse drug events in ambulatory care: a systematic review. *Annals of Pharmacotherapy* 2011; **45**(7–8): 977–89.

49. Miller GC, Britth HC, Valenti L. Adverse drug events in general practice patients in Australia. *Medical Journal of Australia* 2006; **184**(7): 321–4.

50. Barber ND, Alldred DP, Raynor DK et al. Care homes' use of medicines study: prevalence, causes and potential harm of medication errors in care homes for older people. *Quality and Safety in Health Care* 2009; **18**: 341–6.

51. Gurwitz JH, Field TS, Harrold LR et al. Incidence and preventability of adverse drug events among older persons in the ambulatory setting. *JAMA* 2003; **289**(9): 1107–16.

52. Howard RL, Avery AJ, Slavenburg S et al. Which drugs cause preventable admissions to hospital? A systematic review. *British Journal of Clinical Pharmacology* 2007; **63**(2): 136–47.

53. Howard RL, Avery AJ, Howard PD et al. Investigation into the reasons for preventable drug related admissions to a medical admissions unit: observational study. *Quality and Safety in Health Care* 2003; **12**(4): 280–5.

54. Stephens M, Fox B, Kukulka G et al. Medication, allergy, and adverse drug event discrepancies in ambulatory care. *Family Medicine* 2008; **40**(2): 107–10.

55. Doubova Dubova SV, Reyes-Morales H, Torres-Arreola Ldel P et al. Potential drug-drug and drug-disease interactions in prescriptions for ambulatory patients over 50 years of age in family medicine clinics in Mexico City. *BMC Health Services Research* 2007; **7**: 147.

56. McCarthy L, Dolovich L, Haq M et al. Frequency of risk factors that potentially increase harm from medications in older adults receiving primary care. *Canadian Journal of Clinical Pharmacology* 2007; **14**(3): 283–90.

57. Kostopoulou O, Delaney BC, Munro CW. Diagnostic difficulty and error in primary care – a systematic review. *Family Practice* 2008; **25**(6): 400–13.

58. Singh H, Giardina TD, Meyer AN et al. Types and origins of diagnostic errors in primary care settings. *JAMA Internal Medicine* 2013; **173**: 418–25.

59. Casalino LP, Dunham D, Chin MH et al. Frequency of failure to inform patients of clinically significant outpatient test results. *Archives of Internal Medicine* 2009; **169**(12): 1123–9.

60. Cunningham DE, McNab D, Bowie P. Quality and safety issues highlighted by patients in the handling of laboratory test results by general practices – a qualitative study. *BMC Health Services Research* 2014; **14**: 206.

61. Makeham MA, Mira M, Kidd MR. Lessons from the TAPS study – communication failures between hospitals and general practices. *Australian Family Physician* 2008; **37**(9): 735–6.

62. Yu KH, Nation RL, Dooley MJ. Multiplicity of medication safety terms, definitions and functional meanings: when is enough enough? *Quality and Safety in Health Care* 2005; **14**(5): 358–63.

63. LINNEAUS Euro-PC. Learning from International Networks about Errors and Understanding Safety in Primary Care (LINNEAUS Euro-PC) [homepage]. Available at: http://www. linneaus-pc.eu/ (accessed 12 May 2015).

64. Dovey SM, Meyers DS, Phillips RL Jr et al. A preliminary taxonomy of medical errors in family practice. *Quality and Safety in Health Care* 2002; **11**(3): 233–8.

65. Makeham MA, Dovey SM, County M et al. An international taxonomy for errors in general practice: a pilot study. *Medical Journal of Australia* 2002; **177**(2): 68–72.

66. Jacobs S, O'Beirne M, Derfiingher LP et al. Errors and adverse events in family medicine: developing and validating a Canadian taxonomy of errors. *Canadian Family Physician* 2007; **53**(2): 271–6.

67. Buetow S, Kiata L, Liew T et al. Patient error: a preliminary taxonomy. *Annals of Family Medicine* 2009; **7**(3): 223–31.

68. de Wet C, Johnson P, O'Donnell C et al. Can we quantify harm in general practice records? An assessment of precision and power using computer simulation. *BMC Medical Research Methodology* 2013; **13**: 39.

69. Kirk S, Parker D, Claridge T et al. Patient safety culture in primary care: developing a theoretical framework for practical use. *Quality and Safety in Health Care* 2007; **16**(4): 313–20.

70. de Wet C, Spence W, Mash R et al. The development and psychometric evaluation of a safety climate measure for primary care. *Quality and Safety in Health Care* 2010; **19**(6): 578–84.

71. Newham R, Bennie M, Maxwell D et al. Development and psychometric testing of an instrument to measure safety climate perceptions in community pharmacy. *Journal of Evaluation in Clinical Practice* 2014; **20**(6): 1144–52.

72. de Wet C, McKay J, Bowie P. Combining QOF data with the care bundle approach may provide a more meaningful measure of quality in general practice. *BMC Health Services Research* 2012; **12**: 351.

73. de Wet C, O'Donnell C, Bowie P. Developing a preliminary 'never event' list for general practice using consensus-building methods. *British Journal of General Practice* 2014; **64**(620): e159–67.

74. Bowie P, Halley L, Gillies J et al. Searching primary care records for predefined triggers may expose latent risks and adverse events. *Clinical Risk* 2012; **18**(1): 13–18.

75. McKay J, Bradley N, Lough M et al. A review of significant events analysed in general practice: implications for the quality and safety of patient care. *BMC Family Practice* 2009; **10**: 61

76. Bowie P, McNab D, Ferguson J et al. Quality improvement and person-centredness: a participatory mixed methods study to develop the 'always event' concept for primary care. *BMJ Open* 2015; **5**: e0066667.

77. Shekelle, PG, Pronovost PJ, Wachter RM et al. The top patient safety strategies that can be encouraged for adoption now. *Annals of Internal Medicine* 2013; **158**(5 Pt 2): 365–8.

78. Landrigan CP, Parry GJ, Bones CB et al. Temporal trends in rates of patient harm resulting from medical care. *New England Journal of Medicine* 2010; **363**(22): 2124–34.

79. Dovey SM, Wallis KA. Incident reporting in primary care: epidemiology or culture change? *BMJ Quality & Safety* 2011; **20**(12): 1001–3.

80. Royal S, Smeaton L, Avery AJ et al. Interventions in primary care to reduce medication related adverse events and hospital admissions: systematic review and meta-analysis. *Quality and Safety in Health Care* 2006; **15**(1): 23–31.

81. Kwan JL, Lo L, Sampson M, Shojania KG. Medication reconciliation during transitions of care as a patient safety strategy. *Annals of Internal Medicine* 2013; **158**(5 Pt 2): 397–403.

82. Weingart SN, Gandhi TK, Seger AC et al. Patient-reported medication symptoms in primary care. *Archives of Internal Medicine* 2005; **165**(2): 234–40.

83. Zermansky AG, Petty DR, Raynor DK et al. Clinical medication review by a pharmacist of patients on repeat prescriptions in general practice: a randomised controlled trial. *Health Technology Assessment* 2002; **6**(20): 1–86.

84. Scott I. What are the most effective strategies for improving quality and safety of health care? *Internal Medicine Journal* 2009; **39**(6): 389–400.

85. Swinglehurst D, Greenhalgh T, Russell J et al. Receptionist input to quality and safety in repeat prescribing in UK general practice: ethnographic case study. *BMJ* 2011; **343**: d6788.

86. Graham DG, Harris DM, Elder NC et al. Mitigation of patient harm from testing errors in family medicine offices: a report from the American Academy of Family Physicians National Research Network. *Quality and Safety in Health Care* 2008; **17**(3): 201–8.

87. Parnes B, Fernald D, Quintela J et al. Stopping the error cascade: a report on ameliorators from the ASIPS collaborative. *Quality and Safety in Health Care* 2007; **16**(1): 12–16.

88. May C, Finch T, Mair F et al. Understanding the implementation of complex interventions in health care: the normalization process model. *BMC Health Services Research* 2007; **7**: 148.

89. May C, Finch T. Implementation, embedding, and integrating practices: an outline of normalization process theory. *Sociology* 2009; **43**(3): 535–54.

90. Gunn JM, Palmer VJ, Dowrick CF et al. Embedding effective depression care: using theory for primary care organisational and systems change. *Implementation Science* 2010; **5**: 62.

91. Barceló A, Cafiero E, de Boer M et al. Using collaborative learning to improve diabetes care and outcomes: the VIDA project. *Primary Care Diabetes* 2010; **4**(3): 145–53.

92. Youngleson MS, Nkurunziza P, Jennings K et al. Improving a mother to child HIV transmission programme through health system redesign: quality improvement, protocol adjustment and resource addition. *PLoS ONE* 2010; **5**(11): e13891.

93. Franx G, Meeuwissen JA, Sinnema H et al. Quality improvement in depression care in the Netherlands: the depression breakthrough collaborative: a quality improvement report. *International Journal of Integrated Care* 2009; **9**: e84.

94. Humphreys J, Harvey G, Coleiro M et al. A collaborative project to improve identification and management of patients with chronic kidney disease in a primary care setting in Greater Manchester. *BMJ Quality & Safety* 2012; **21**(8): 700–8.

95. Scott I, Phelps G. Measurement for improvement: getting one to follow the other. *Internal Medicine Journal* 2009; **39**(6): 347–51.

96. Siriwardena AN. Quality improvement projects for appraisal and revalidation of general practitioners. *Quality in Primary Care* 2011; **19**(4): 205–9.

97. House of Commons Health Committee. How many NHS GP consultations are estimated to have taken place in each year from 1995? [UK Parliament Commons Select Committee

record]. 2010. Available at: http://www.publications.parliament.uk/pa/cm200910/cmselect/cmhealth/269/269we46.htm (accessed 12 May 2015).

98. Wachter RM, Pronovost PJ, Shekelle PG. Strategies to improve patient safety: the evidence base matures. *Annals of Internal Medicine* 2013; **158**: 350–2.

99. Is primary-care research a lost cause? *Lancet* 2003; **361**(9362): 977.

100. Mid Staffordshire NHS Foundation Trust Public Inquiry. *Report of the Mid Staffordshire NHS Foundation Trust Public Inquiry: Executive Summary.* HC 947. Norwich: The Stationery Office (TSO), 2013. Available at: http://www.ajustnhs.com/wp-content/uploads/2012/06/Francis-Executive-summary.pdf (accessed 25 May 2015).

101. WHO. *The World Health Report 2008: Primary Health Care; Now More than Ever.* Geneva: WHO, 2008. Available at: http://www.who.int/whr/2008/whr08_en.pdf (accessed 27 November 2015).

102. Hummers-Pradier E, Beyer M, Chevallier P et al. The Research Agenda for General Practice / Family Medicine and Primary Health Care in Europe: part 1; background and methodology. *European Journal of General Practice* 2009; **15**(4): 243–50.

103. Van Royen P, Beyer M, Chevallier P et al. Series: The Research Agenda for General Practice/Family Medicine and Primary Health Care in Europe: part 6; reaction on commentaries – how to continue with the Research Agenda? *European Journal of General Practice* 2011; **17**(1): 58–61.

104. Reuben DB, Tinetti ME. Goal-oriented patient care – an alternative health outcomes paradigm. *New England Journal of Medicine* 2012; **366**: 777–9.

105. Lionis C, Shea S, Markaki A. Introducing and implementing a compassionate care elective for medical students in Crete. *Journal of Holistic Healthcare* 2011; **8**(3): 38–41.

106. Waddington C, Egger D; WHO Working Group on Service Delivery. *Integrated Health Care Services: What and Why?* Technical Brief No. 1. Geneva: WHO, 2008. Available at: http://www.who.int/healthsystems/technical_brief_final.pdf (accessed 27 November 2015).

107. Frampton SB, Guastello S, Lepore M. Compassion as the foundation of patient-centered care: the importance of compassion in action. *Journal of Comparative Effectiveness Research* 2013; **2**(5): 443–55.

108. Lionis, C, Shea S. Encouraging a focus on compassionate care within general practice/family medicine. In: Shea S, Wynyard R, Lionis C, editors. *Providing Compassionate Healthcare: Challenges in Policy and Practice.* Abingdon and New York: Routledge, 2014. pp. 103–16.

109. Shea S, Wynyard R, Lionis C. Introduction. In: Shea S, Wynyard R, Lionis C, editors. *Providing Compassionate Healthcare: Challenges in Policy and Practice.* Abingdon and New York: Routledge. pp. 1–6.

110. Mercer SW, Smith SM, Wyke S et al. Multimorbidity in primary care: developing the research agenda. *Family Practice* 2009; **26**(2): 79–80.

111. Gill TM, Gahbauer EA, Allore HG et al. Transitions between frailty states among community-living older persons. *Archives of Internal Medicine* 2006; **166**(4): 418–23.

112. Ensrud KE, Ewing SK, Taylor BC et al; Study of Osteoporotic Fractures Research Group. Frailty and risk of falls, fracture, and mortality in older women: the study of osteoporotic fractures. *Journals of Gerontology: Series A; Biological Sciences and Medical Sciences* 2007; **62**: 744–51.

113. Langan J, Mercer SW, Smith DJ. Multimorbidity and mental health: can psychiatry rise to the challenge? *British Journal of Psychiatry* 2013; **202**(6): 391–3.

114. Akner G. Analysis of multimorbidity in individual elderly nursing home residents: development of a multimorbidity matrix. *Archives of Gerontology and Geriatrics* 2009; **49**(3): 413–19.

115. Agency for Healthcare Research and Quality (AHRQ). *The Patient-Centered Medical Home: Strategies to put Patients at the Centre of Primary Care.* Publication no. AHRQ 11-0029. Rockville, MD: AHRQ, 2011. Available at: https://pcmh.ahrq.gov/sites/default/files/attach ments/Strategies%20to%20Put%20Patients%20at%20the%20Center%20of%20Primary%20 Care.pdf (accessed 25 November 2015).

116. INVOLVE. What is public involvement in research? Available at: http://www.invo.org.uk/ find-out-more/what-is-public-involvement-in-research-2/ (accessed 25 November 2015).

117. Department of Health. *Department of Health: Departmental Report 2006.* Cm 6814. Norwich: TSO, 2006. Available at: https://www.gov.uk/government/uploads/system/uploads/attachment _data/file/272276/6814.pdf(accessed on 1 February 2015).

118. Fraser Health Authority. *Community Engagement Framework.* Vancouver: Fraser Health Authority, 2009. Available at: http://www.fraserhealth.ca/media/Community%20Engagement %20Framework.pdf (accessed 9 September 2015).

119. Patient-Centered Outcomes Research Institute (PCORI). About us. Available at: http://www. pcori.org/about-us (accessed 25 November 2015).

120. PCORI. *Patient-Centred Outcomes Research Definition Revision: Response to Public Input; Consensus Definition as of February 15, 2012.* Washington DC: PCORI, 2012. Available at: http://www.pcori.org/assets/PCOR-Definition-Revised-Draft-and-Responses-to-Input.pdf (accessed on 1 February 2015).

121. Starfield B, Shi L, Macinko J. Contribution of primary care to health systems and health. *Milbank Quarterly* 2005; **83**(3): 457–502.

122. Franks P, Fiscella K. Primary care physicians and specialists as personal physicians: health care expenditures and mortality experience. *Journal of Family Practice* 1998; **47**(2): 105–9.

123. Starfield B. Primary care and health: a cross-national comparison. *JAMA* 1991; **266**(16): 2268–71.

124. Starfield B. Is primary care essential? *Lancet* 1994; **344**(8930): 1129–33.

125. Gulliford MC. Availability of primary care doctors and population health in England: is there an association? *Journal of Public Health* 2002; **24**(4): 252–4.

126. Shi L. The relationship between primary care and life chances. *Journal of Health Care for the Poor and Underserved* 1992; **3**(2): 321–35.

127. Shi L. Primary care, specialty care, and life chances. *International Journal of Health Services* 1994; **24**(3): 431–58.

128. Vogel RL, Ackermann RJ. Is primary care physician supply correlated with health outcomes? *International Journal of Health Services* 1998; **28**(1): 183–96.

129. Shi L, Macinko J, Starfield B et al. The relationship between primary care, income inequality, and mortality in US States, 1980–1995. *Journal of the American Board of Family Practice* 2003; **16**(5): 412–22.

130. Manuel DG, Maaten S, Thiruchelvam D et al. Primary care in the health care system. In: Jaakkimainen L, Upshur RE, Klein-Geltink JE et al., editors. *Primary Care in Ontario: ICES Atlas.* Toronto: Institute for Clinical Evaluative Sciences, 2006. pp. 1–14. Available at: http:// www.ices.on.ca/Publications/Atlases-and-Reports/2006/Primary-care-in-Ontario.aspx (accessed 27 November 2015).

131. Parchman ML, Burge SK. The patient-physician relationship, primary care attributes, and preventive services. *Family Medicine* 2004; **36**(1): 22–7.

132. Rosenblatt RA, Wright GE, Baldwin LM et al. The effect of the doctor-patient relationship on emergency department use among the elderly. *American Journal of Public Health* 2000; **90**(1): 97–102.

133. Mainous AG 3rd, Gill JM. The importance of continuity of care in the likelihood of future hospitalization: is site of care equivalent to a primary clinician? *American Journal of Public Health* 1998; **88**(10): 1539–41.

134. Weiss LJ, Blustein J. Faithful patients: the effect of long-term physician-patient relationships on the costs and use of health care by older Americans. *American Journal of Public Health* 1996; **86**(12): 1742–7.

135. Roos NP. Who should do the surgery? Tonsillectomy-adenoidectomy in one Canadian province. *Inquiry* 1979; **16**(1): 73–83.

136. Forrest CB, Starfield B. The effect of first-contact care with primary care clinicians on ambulatory health care expenditures. *Journal of Family Practice* 1996; **43**(1): 40–8.

137. Greenfield S, Nelson EC, Zubkoff M et al. Variations in resource utilization among medical specialties and systems of care: results from the medical outcomes study. *JAMA* 1992; **267**(12): 1624–30.

138. Stewart M. Towards a global definition of patient centred care. *BMJ* 2001; **322**(7284): 444–5.

139. Mead N, Bower P. Patient-centredness: a conceptual framework and review of the empirical literature. *Social Science and Medicine* 2000; **51**(7): 1087–110.

140. Kovess-Masfety V, Saragoussi D, Sevilla-Dedieu C et al. What makes people decide who to turn to when faced with a mental health problem? Results from a French survey. *BMC Public Health* 2007; **7**: 188.

141. Fiscella K, Meldrum S, Franks P et al. Patient trust: is it related to patient-centered behavior of primary care physicians? *Medical Care* 2004; **42**(11): 1049–55.

142. Sweeney K. Personal knowledge. *BMJ* 2006; **332**(7534): 129–30.

143. Chande VT, Kinnane JM. Role of the primary care provider in expediting care of children with acute appendicitis. *Archives of Pediatrics and Adolescent Medicine* 1996; **150**(7): 703–6.

144. Bindman AB, Grumbach K, Osmond D et al. Primary care and receipt of preventive services. *Journal of General Internal Medicine* 1996; **11**(5): 269–76.

145. Shea S, Misra D, Ehrlich MH et al. Predisposing factors for severe, uncontrolled hypertension in an inner-city minority population. *New England Journal of Medicine* 1992; **327**(11): 776–81.

146. Starfield B, Shi L. Policy relevant determinants of health: an international perspective. *Health Policy* 2002; **60**(3): 201–18.

147. Whittle J, Lin CJ, Lave JR et al. Relationship of provider characteristics to outcomes, process, and costs of care for community-acquired pneumonia. *Medical Care* 1998; **36**(7): 977–87.

148. Rosser WW. Approach to diagnosis by primary care clinicians and specialists: is there a difference? *Journal of Family Practice* 1996; **42**(2): 139–44.

149. Richards DA, Toop LJ, Epton MJ et al. Home management of mild to moderately severe community-acquired pneumonia: a randomised controlled trial. *Medical Journal of Australia* 2005; **183**(5): 235–8.

150. Starfield B, Gérvas J, Mangin D. Clinical care and health disparities. *Annual Review of Public Health* 2012; **33**: 89–106.

151. Basu J, Clancy C. Racial disparity, primary care, and specialty referral. *Health Services Research* 2001; **36**(6 Pt 2): 64–77.

152. Hogg W, Rowan M, Russell G et al. Framework for primary care organizations: the importance of a structural domain. *International Journal for Quality in Health Care* 2008; **20**(5): 308–13.

153. Shi L, Starfield B, Xu J. Validating the Adult Primary Care Assessment Tool. *Journal of Family Practice* 2001; **50**(161): 161W–75W.

154. Campbell SM, Roland MO, Buetow SA. Defining quality of care. *Social Science & Medicine* 2000; **51**(11): 1611–25.

155. Starfield B, Mangin D. An international perspective on the basis of pay-for-performance. In: Gillam S, Siriwardena AN, editors. *The Quality and Outcomes Framework: QOF – Transforming General Practice.* Oxford: Radcliffe, 2011. pp. 147–55.

156. Van Herck P, De Smedt D, Annemans L et al. Systematic review: effects, design choices, and context of pay-for-performance in health care. *BMC Health Services Research* 2010; **10**: 247.

157. Campbell SM, Reeves D, Kontopantelis E et al. Effects of pay for performance on the quality of primary care in England. *New England Journal of Medicine* 2009; **361**(4): 368–78.

158. Doran T, Kontopantelis E, Valderas JM et al. Effect of financial incentives on incentivised and non-incentivised clinical activities: longitudinal analysis of data from the UK Quality and Outcomes Framework. *BMJ* 2011; **342**: d3590.

159. Kontopantelis E, Reeves D, Valderas JM et al. Recorded quality of primary care for patients with diabetes in England before and after the introduction of a financial incentive scheme: a longitudinal observational study. *BMJ Quality & Safety* 2013; **22**(1): 53–64.

160. Gillam SJ, Siriwardena AN, Steel N. Pay-for-performance in the United Kingdom: impact of the Quality and Outcomes Framework; a systematic review. *Annals of Family Medicine* 2012; **10**(5): 461–8.

161. Kontopantelis E, Springate DA, Ashworth M et al. Investigating the relationship between quality of primary care and premature mortality in England: a spatial whole-population study. *BMJ* 2015; **350**: h904.

162. Sutton M, Nikolova S, Boaden R et al. Reduced mortality with hospital pay for performance in England. *New England Journal of Medicine* 2012; **367**(19): 1821–8.

163. Calderón-Larrañaga A, Soljak M, Cecil E et al. Does higher quality of primary healthcare reduce hospital admissions for diabetes complications? A national observational study. *Diabetic Medicine* 2014; **31**(6): 657–65.

164. Soljak M, Calderon-Larrañaga A, Sharma P et al. Does higher quality primary health care reduce stroke admissions? A national cross-sectional study. British Journal of General Practice 2011; 61(593): e801–7.

165. Lester H, Schmittdiel J, Selby J et al. The impact of removing financial incentives from clinical quality indicators: longitudinal analysis of four Kaiser Permanente indicators. *BMJ.* 2010; **340**: c1898.

166. Villalbí JR, Guarga A, Pasarín MI et al. [An evaluation of the impact of primary care reform on health] [Spanish]. *Atención Primaria* 1999; **24**(8): 468–74.

167. Barros FC, Matijasevich A, Requejo JH et al. Recent trends in maternal, newborn, and child health in Brazil: progress toward Millennium Development Goals 4 and 5. *American Journal of Public Health* 2010; **100**(10): 1877–9.

168. Macinko J, Guanais FC, de Fatima M et al. Evaluation of the impact of the Family Health Program on infant mortality in Brazil, 1990–2002. *Journal of Epidemiology and Community Health* 2006; **60**(1): 13–19.

169. Szwarcwald CL, Souza-Júnior PR, Damacena GN. Socioeconomic inequalities in the use of outpatient services in Brazil according to health care need: evidence from the World Health Survey. *BMC Health Services Research* 2010; **10**: 217.

170. Yiengprugsawan V, Carmichael GA, Lim LL et al. Has universal health insurance reduced socioeconomic inequalities in urban and rural health service use in Thailand? *Health & Place* 2010; **16**(5): 1030–7.

171. Suraratdecha C, Saithanu S, Tangcharoensathien V. Is universal coverage a solution for disparities in health care? Findings from three low-income provinces of Thailand. *Health Policy* 2005; **73**(3): 272–84.

172. Tangcharoensathien V, Wibulpholprasert S, Nitayaramphong S. Knowledge-based changes to health systems: the Thai experience in policy development. *Bulletin of the World Health Organization* 2004; **82**(10): 750–6.

173. Salisbury C, Johnson L, Purdy S et al. Epidemiology and impact of multimorbidity in primary care: a retrospective cohort study. *British Journal of General Practice* 2011; **61**(582): e12–21.

174. Barnett K, Mercer SW, Norbury M et al. Epidemiology of multimorbidity and implications for health care, research, and medical education: a cross-sectional study. *Lancet* 2012; **380**(9836): 37–43.

175. Wang HH, Wang JJ, Wong SY et al. Epidemiology of multimorbidity in China and implications for the healthcare system: cross-sectional survey among 162,464 community household residents in southern China. *BMC Medicine* 2014; **12**: 188.

176. Mangin D, Heath I, Jamoulle M. Beyond diagnosis: responding to the comorbidity challenge *BMJ* 2012; **44**: e3526.

177. WHO. *Monitoring the Building Blocks of Health Systems: A Handbook of Indicators and Their Measurement Strategies.* Geneva: WHO, 2010. Available at: http://www.who.int/healthinfo/systems/WHO_MBHSS_2010_full_web.pdf (accessed 27 November 2015).

178. Organisation for Economic Co-operation and Development (OECD), Eurostat, WHO. *A System of Health Accounts.* Paris: OECD Publishing, 2011. Available at: http://www.who.int/health-accounts/methodology/sha2011.pdf (accessed 27 November 2015).

179. Kringos D, Boerma W, Bourgueil Y et al. The strength of primary care in Europe: an international comparative study. *British Journal of General Practice* 2013; **63**(616): e742–50.

180. Saksena P, Xu K, Evans DB. *Impact of Out-Of-Pocket Payments for Treatment of Non-Communicable Diseases in Developing Countries: A Review of Literature.* Discussion Paper No. 2. Geneva: WHO, 2011. Available at: http://www.who.int/health_financing/documents/dp_e_11_02-ncd_finburden.pdf?ua=1 (accessed 27 November 2015).

181. OECD. *Health at a Glance 2013: OECD Indicators.* Paris: OECD Publishing, 2013. Available at: http://www.oecd.org/els/health-systems/Health-at-a-Glance-2013.pdf (accessed 27 November 2015).

182. Thomson S, Foubister T, Mossialos E. Can user charges make health care more efficient? *BMJ* 2010; **341**: c3759.

183. Xu K, Evans DB, Kawabata K et al. Household catastrophic health expenditure: a multicountry analysis. *Lancet* 2003; **362**(9378): 111–17.

184. International Conference on Primary Health Care. *Declaration of Alma-Ata: International Conference on Primary Health Care, Alma-Ata, USSR, 6–12 September 1978.* Alma-Ata: WHO, 1978. Available at: http://www.who.int/publications/almaata_declaration_en.pdf (accessed 27 November 2015).

185. Donaldson MS, Yordy KD, Vanselow NA, editors; Institute of Medicine Division of Health Care Services Committee on the Future of Primary Care, author. *Defining Primary Care: An Interim Report.* Washington DC: National Academy Press, 1994.

186. Kruk ME, Porignon D, Rockers PC et al. The contribution of primary care to health and health systems in low- and middle-income countries: a critical review of major primary care initiatives. *Social Science & Medicine* 2010; **70**(6): 904–11.

187. De Maeseneer J, van Weel C, Egilman D et al. Strengthening primary care: addressing the disparity between vertical and horizontal investment. *British Journal of General Practice* 2008; **58**(546): 3–4.

188. Marchal B, Cavalli A, Kegels G. Global health actors claim to support health system strengthening—is this reality or rhetoric? *PLoS Medicine* 2009; **6**(4): e1000059.

189. Dye C, Boerma T, Evans D et al. *The World Health Report 2013: Research for Universal Health Coverage.* Geneva: WHO, 2013. Available at: http://apps.who.int/iris/bitstream/10665/85761/2/9789240690837_eng.pdf (accessed 27 November 2015).

190. United Nations (UN) Department of Economic and Social Affairs Division for Sustainable Development. Open Working Group proposal for sustainable development goals. New York, NY: UN Department of Economic and Social Affairs, n.d. Available at: https://sustainabledevelopment.un.org/sdgsproposal (accessed 27 November 2015).

191. Evans DB, Elovainio R, Humphreys G et al. *The World Health Report: Health Systems Financing; The Path to Universal Coverage.* Geneva: WHO, 2010. Available at: http://www.who.int/entity/whr/2010/whr10_en.pdf?ua=1 (accessed 27 November 2015).

192. Gosden T, Forland F, Kristiansen I et al. Capitation, salary, fee-for-service and mixed systems of payment: effects on the behaviour of primary care physicians. *Cochrane Database of Systematic Reviews* 2000;(3):CD002215.

193. Scott A, Sivey P, Ait Ouakrim D et al. The effect of financial incentives on the quality of health care provided by primary care physicians. *Cochrane Database of Systematic Reviews* 2011; (9): CD008451.

194. Lagarde M, Haines A, Palmer N. The impact of conditional cash transfers on health outcomes and use of health services in low and middle income countries. *Cochrane Database of Systematic Reviews* 2009; 4(4): CD008137.

195. Swanwick T, McKimm J. What is clinical leadership ... and why is it important? *Clinical Teacher* 2011; **8**(1): 22–6.

196. Scally G, Donaldson LJ. Clinical governance and the drive for quality improvement in the new NHS in England. *BMJ* 1998; **317**(7150): 61–5.

197. Parsons S, Winterbottom A, Cross P et al. *The Quality of Patient Engagement and Involvement in Primary Care: An Inquiry into the Quality of General Practice in England.* London: The King's Fund, 2010.

198. Carman KL, Dardess P, Maurer M et al. Patient and family engagement: a framework for understanding the elements and developing interventions and policies. *Health Affairs* 2013; **32**(2): 223–31.

199. Glasser M, Pathman D. Renewed focus on primary health care (PHC). *Education for Health* 2009; **22**(3): 429.

200. Frenk J, Chen L, Bhutta ZA et al. Health professionals for a new century: transforming education to strengthen health systems in an interdependent world. *Lancet* 2010; **376**(9756): 1923–58.

201. The Network: Towards Unity for Health [homepage]. Available at: www.the-networktufh.org/ (accessed 3 September 2015).

202. Training for Health Equity Network (THEnet) [homepage]. Available at: http://thenetcommunity.org/ (accessed 3 September 2015).

203. WHO. *Transforming and Scaling Up Health Professionals' Education and Training: World Health Organization Guidelines 2013.* Geneva: WHO, 2013. Available at: http://apps.who.int/iris/bitstream/10665/93635/1/9789241506502_eng.pdf (accessed 27 November 2015).

204. Nkomazana O, Peersman W, Willcox M et al. Human resources for health in Botswana: the results of in-country database and reports analysis. *Afr J Prm Health Care Fam Med* 2014; **6**(1), Art. #716, 8 pages. Available at http://dx.doi.org/10.4102/phcfm.v6i1.716.

205. Nkomazana O, Mash R, Shaibu S et al. Stakeholders' perceptions on shortage of healthcare workers in primary healthcare in Botswana: Focus group discussions. *PLoS ONE* 2015; **10**(8): e0135846. doi:10.1371/journal. pone.0135846.

206. Baum F, MacDougall C, Smith D. Participatory action research. *Journal of Epidemiology & Community Health* 2006; **60**(10): 854–7.

207. Mash B, Meulenberg-Buskens I. 'Holding it lightly': the co-operative inquiry group; a method for developing educational materials. *Medical Education* 2001; **35**(12): 1108–14.

208. Nkomazana O, Mash R, Phaladze N. Understanding the organisational culture of district health services: Mahalapye and Ngamiland health districts of Botswana. *Afr J Prm Health Care Fam Med.* 2015; **7**(1), Art. #907, 9 pages. Available at http://dx.doi. org/10.4102/phcfm. v7i1.907 (accessed 5 February 2016)

209. Human resources for primary health care in Africa – HURAPRIM. *Why Uganda needs to increase its health budget: A briefing for MPs.* 2015. Available at www.huraprim.ugent. be/drupal/?q=dissemination/why-uganda-needs-increase-its-health-budget-briefing-mps (accessed 5 February 2016).

210. 'newsroom editor'. Supporting family practice in Africa. Brussels and Luxembourg: European Commission, 19 May 2015. Available at: http://ec.europa.eu/programmes/horizon2020/en/news/supporting-family-practice-africa (accessed 3 September 2015).

211. Niederkrotenthaler T, Dorner TE, Maier M. Development of a practical tool to measure the impact of publications on the society based on focus group discussions with scientists. *BMC Public Health* 2011; **11**: 588.

212. van Driel ML, Maier M, De Maeseneer J. Measuring the impact of family medicine research: scientific citations or societal impact? *Family Practice* 2007; **24**(5): 401–2.

SECTION III

Commissioning of primary care research

Introduction

....

Bob Mash

Despite the importance of strengthening primary healthcare, the global funding agenda is often not well aligned with the burden of disease and the needs of society in different countries. There may be more of a focus on specific diseases and technologies than on strengthening health services and systems. In many parts of the world, the primary care researchers are also not sufficiently established to compete for global funds, and local governments may not prioritise health research in general or primary care research in particular.

This section of the book explores the many factors that may influence the commissioning and funding of primary care research. We have juxtaposed the views of researchers with the viewpoint of potential funders, and give an example of how Australia has been successfully championing primary care research.

CHAPTER 13

Primary care research: how to put local priorities into a world led by global funding

. . . .

Leslie London

INTRODUCTION

In 1990, the Commission on Health Research for Development coined the term '90:10 gap' to capture the mismatch between research funding and health priorities globally, arguing that 90% of research funding globally went to address 10% of the extant burden of disease.[1] Has this disparity changed in recent years with the growth of major international funders, seemingly committed to addressing the needs of poor countries, including the World Bank; The Global Fund for the eradication of TB, AIDS and malaria; the Bill & Melinda Gates Foundation; and the International AIDS Vaccine Initiative?[2] Some have argued that the new institutional environment has generated problems of its own, related to the lack of accountability of these large funders and to their impacts on national health systems.[3] For example, Sridhar points out that new funding for global health has largely been in the form of discretionary funding focused on a specific disease priority and reliant on a third party for implementation.[2] Such funding does not provide for building sustainable health systems or flexibility in local priority setting.

Moreover, there is strong evidence of donors influencing research agendas in health. In reviewing health systems and policy research (HSPR) conducted in low- and middle-income countries (LMICs) between 2000 and 2002, Gonzales-Block showed that the pattern of research coincided with the preferences of donors.[4] Topics most commonly chosen included 'disease burden', whereas the least likely foci included topics such as 'equity' and 'economic policy and health'. The author argued that, in the field of HSPR, donors determine research priorities, and called for national and international consensus to ensure that different stakeholders' agendas play a complementary rather than defining role in support of health system objectives.

Further, traditional multilateral organisations supporting health research, such as the World Health Organization (WHO) and UNICEF, have been eclipsed in this funding environment in which multiple bilateral financing mechanisms, involving a few powerful governments partnering with philanthropic foundations and non-governmental organisations, have realigned the objectives of these multilateral organisations to match their own agendas. This allows powerful governments to use funding mechanisms as a way to define a separate mandate and to push specific goals.[4]

PRIMARY CARE RESEARCH IN LOW- AND MIDDLE-INCOME COUNTRIES

Notwithstanding the global context for health research, for healthcare professionals working in primary care, health research can still play a key role in improving the quality of care, enhancing the responsiveness of services and informing outreach and prevention, as well as promoting the articulation of primary care services with other levels and components of the health service and with sectors outside health whose mandates broadly address the social determinants of health. Relevant primary care research is often best accomplished by qualitative or mixed methods, though randomised controlled trials in primary care settings are not uncommon to establish evidence of effectiveness. Yet it would be an understatement to say that it is harder to attract grant funding for studies that are not quantitative in approach or biomedical in framing. Moreover, many of the most burdensome problems in primary care are those that struggle to find their place in research agendas informed by quantitative priority-setting processes because of low visibility and traction. For example, lack of funding for mental health research, despite its contribution to burden of disease, has been widely noted in developed countries[5–7] all the more neglected in LMICs.[8]

Moreover, health services research and health systems research are intuitively the rubrics under which research for improving primary care would be best located. Yet despite a growing interest in these fields,[9] it is still the case that the majority of funding for health research is driven by interest in biomedical solutions and technological fixes. For example, the recipients of the Gates Foundation Grand Challenges in Global Health over the past decade include only one study that might be said to be research with an explicit health systems–strengthening perspective; rather, the vast majority of Grand Challenge funding is devoted to golden-bullet technological solutions to health problems. Of the 91 Global Health projects funded since the challenge began, 29 studies were devoted to identifying new biomarkers for health and disease states and 23 to vaccine studies, reflecting the singular view that new technological advances are key to meeting global health challenges.

The following two case studies further explore the mismatch between funding investments and what is needed in LMICs to improve primary care.

LIBERIA AND EBOLA

Liberia is one of the poorest countries in the world. It survived a debilitating and protracted civil war that witnessed some of the worst atrocities against civilians in the twentieth century. Its gradual recovery and fledgling efforts to establish a functional health system received scant research attention from global funders of health research until the Ebola outbreak in 2014. Indeed, if one does a PubMed search on 'Liberia' *and* 'Ebola', one will find all but four of the 142 articles identified (i.e. 97%) were published after the start of the 2014 outbreak. In contrast, if one repeats the PubMed search but uses the search terms 'Liberia' *and* 'health systems', one will find only 28 articles, the majority of which (68%) precede the Ebola epidemic. Of the more recent citations, most are related to the Ebola epidemic but are commentaries rather than empirical studies involving health systems research.

Ironically, in July 2014, just as the epidemic was emerging in West Africa, Svoronos and colleagues published an analysis of rural Liberians' confidence in healthcare with the title 'Can the health system deliver?'[10] Their analysis found that, overall, there was low confidence in the healthcare system, that poor experiences of past visits shaped low expectations of access to future care and that confidence was inversely related to education and socio-economic status. Yet it is now widely recognised that part of the reason for the difficulty in controlling the Ebola outbreak in the region was widespread distrust among rural populations of 'Western' healthcare, perceived to be associated with spreading the disease rather than containing it. Perhaps if only one-twentieth of the funding poured into massive investigations into new drugs and vaccines for Ebola had been made available earlier to identify how best to strengthen core public health functions – such as community participation and ownership – the Ebola epidemic might have been contained without the widespread loss of life that has now occurred in the region.

Other authors have commented on the role of the upstream economic policy context as a determinant for the failure to contain the epidemic in West Africa – for example, through structural adjustment and neoliberal market policies undermining health systems, in the failure to translate economic growth into services for the poor[11] and in the deforestation led by logging companies that has changed the natural habitat of the bat vectors for Ebola.[12] Indeed, Liberia has one of the highest foreign direct investment to gross domestic product ratios in the world, based upon a plethora of concession agreements with numerous transnational corporations (TNCs) and has posted economic growth rates of in excess of 5% in the last decade yet has failed to lift its population out of poverty or to achieve anything near its health Millennium Development Goals (MDGs).[13] As argued by the People's Health Movement, these are the social and economic roots of the Ebola epidemic, serious consideration of which would 'force the rich and the powerful – global leaders, the capitalist press, the institutions of capitalism, the captains of industry both nationally and globally, UN [United Nations] agencies – to confront the reality of Africa's poverty and inequality'.[12] Yet current investments in health research related to Ebola steer well clear of addressing upstream determinants. Indeed, if one examines the projects funded by Gates Grand

Challenges in Global Health, not one of the 1689 research projects funded since inception has been located in Guinea, Liberia or Sierra Leone, the countries now at the epicentre of the recent Ebola epidemic.

HEALTH RESEARCH IN THE WESTERN CAPE PROVINCE OF SOUTH AFRICA

A second example of the dominance of a few small global funders in health research and their influence over the health research agenda is illustrated in a review of health research conducted in the Western Cape Province of South Africa during 2011 and 2012.[14] The study found that, while just over 50% of research studies conducted on the platform were at district level, there was an overwhelming preponderance of studies and of grant funding (about 65%) focused on HIV and TB, to the detriment of studies addressing mental health, injury, non-communicable disease and nutrition, despite the major contribution made by these risk factors and conditions to the local burden of disease.[15] Moreover, the bulk of research funding was contributed to by a handful of very big global funders – particularly in the areas of HIV and TB. South African government funding comprised only about 8% of health research funding. It is difficult to ensure that local priorities can be met if 90% of research funding comes from outside sources.

LMICs have been challenged to increase government allocations to research and development with a target proposed by WHO of 2% of health budgets earmarked for supporting health research. There are examples of LMICs successfully achieving this target. Brazil, for example, allocated 4.15% of its health budget between 2000 and 2002 to supporting health research and has managed to institute a process of monitoring and evaluation of research activities to align health research with national priorities.[16]

CONCLUSION

What these two cases suggest is that (1) the research agenda for LMICs is often shaped by forces far beyond the control of national governments, and (2) the structural and social determinants of health and diseases remain the poor orphans of global health research. Yet it is precisely this kind of research that is likely to strengthen health systems to be able to prevent, contain or treat epidemic, endemic and emerging diseases. That national sovereignty is important in setting research priorities is not a matter of parochial interest or an appeal to a more just and fair world; it is also increasingly being recognised as essential for a more effective global health architecture in which global health priorities should be shaped by country-level priorities if scale-up of interventions is to achieve the MDGs.[17]

The mismatch between burden of disease priorities and the actual research agenda for a country is a problem reported commonly in developing countries where donor agendas have set the pattern of research.[18] Moreover, the major investments in global health research appear to continue to focus on disease-specific priorities and lack a health systems perspective. Ironically, South Africa, Liberia, Sierra Leone and Guinea, as the country case studies discussed in this chapter, have one thing in common – they have all ratified the International Covenant of Economic Social and Cultural Rights (ICESCR). Besides its provision for the right to enjoy 'the highest attainable standard of ... health' (Article 12), Article 15 of the ICESCR affords anyone the right 'to enjoy the benefits of scientific progress'.[19] Yet if the direction of scientific inquiry is essentially determined by the chequebooks of the biggest funders, there is no guarantee that research will address key but unfashionable research areas or invest in studies using methods not popular with large global funders. As a result, it would be unlikely that scientific research emerging from such a milieu would necessarily meet the needs of the most vulnerable in the best possible ways. However, it is precisely at the interface between communities and the health services, at primary care level, that health research might deliver the best likelihood of sharing the benefits of scientific progress with those who need it most.

CHAPTER 14

Primary healthcare and international development assistance

. . . .

Robert Fryatt

In the year 2000, countries all around the world signed up to some ambitious Millennium Development Goals (MGDs), with targets to be met by 2015. Health targets for maternal and child health and communicable diseases (in particular, HIV, TB and malaria) featured large among these goals. The final report cards for many countries have still to be completed, but already there is general agreement that the goals helped galvanise international and national support in many low- and middle-income countries of Africa and that many countries have seen remarkable improvements.[20] However, there are still too many countries in which progress is poor and uneven and major inequities are seemingly getting worse in many countries. The lead up to the MDGs has again led to considerable debate about the role and effectiveness of international development assistance. Its significance is undoubtedly waning, given the rising economies of many low- and middle-income countries, the increase in importance of south–south cooperation, especially from China, and the increase in flows of private sector investments. However, the sums involved, estimated at US$31.3 billion in 2013,[21] remain significant, and debates continue about how these funds might be better used in the post-MDG era, with a move to health-related Sustainable Development Goals (SDGs).[22]

The MDG era has been dominated by international investments in developing countries aimed at reducing the problems of HIV, TB and malaria and, in recent years, improving maternal, neonatal and child health services. There seems to have been little appetite for investing in comprehensive primary healthcare (PHC) directly, despite constant reminders from world leaders as to its importance. *The World Health Report 2008* focused on the need for PHC, making clear the dangers of the current trend for fragmented investments in a health system.[23] The report was accompanied by arguments to redirect disease-specific funds to PHC investments.[24] However, this shift has not yet happened, and the focus of many of the health-related SDGs are, as before, with the continuation of many of the previous goals and the introduction of new disease-specific goals, such as for hepatitis.

However, there is also now a call for universal health coverage (UHC) to be one of SDGs, with PHC and integrated service delivery featuring large in the global discussion on how UHC might be realised in many countries. An opportunity is again arising for PHC. Lessons from the past can show how this opportunity can be best used to get international investment to support national efforts to strengthen PHC services.

First, international donors need to be able to measure results and, increasingly, want to know how many people have benefitted, and where, with simple messages that can be relayed to parliaments and taxpayers in donor countries. Investing in health system strengthening or primary healthcare is not sufficient unless backed up by good evidence of health workers and facilities serving communities who were previously deprived of basic, essential services and evidence that this is leading to better health.

Secondly, mechanisms for investing international resources and delivering these results need to be efficient, transparent and with clear accountability mechanisms to ensure funds go where they are meant to.[25] Experience has shown that investments can be more efficient when they support existing country systems and have monitoring and evaluation mechanisms aligned with national efforts. For PHC, this can be difficult due to there being no one area for investment. Traditionally, funds go to the development of certain aspects of PHC, such as the human workforce; access to essential drugs, nutrition, water and sanitation; or building demand and community systems through non-government agencies. A vehicle for comprehensive investment is often lacking.

Thirdly, international investments are effective when responding to demand and existing national efforts. For international investments to support PHC, there has to be a strong articulation of what is required at national level. Countries such as Ethiopia and Rwanda have been very successful in using the grants from The Global Fund; Gavi, the Vaccine Alliance; and many bilateral donors to build their PHC services through strong leadership, effective planning and strong, inclusive monitoring and evaluation.

So, as we move into the new post-MDG era, there is already clear recognition of the importance of PHC in delivering UHC, and many international donors are now open to assisting national stakeholders in developing their PHC services. There is much that those advocating for more PHC investment can do. Some suggested priorities are provided here.

CREATE STRONG NATIONAL PRIMARY HEALTHCARE AGENDAS AND LEADERSHIP TO ATTRACT INTERNATIONAL INVESTMENT

Obviously, the government policy on PHC is key, as is the national leadership that can speak to the importance of it for each country. Also important, though, is the evidence that there are ways to invest in PHC and deliver results and that groups exist who are willing to take risks and expand PHC services into underserved areas, with good collaboration across the many professions required to deliver an effective PHC service.

WORK WITH THE INTERNATIONAL COMMUNITY TO AGREE UNIVERSAL, COMPOSITE MEASURES OF SUCCESS

The proposed measures for UHC cover the delivery of many services that can only be efficiently delivered through an effective PHC system. These composite measures of UHC are an opportunity to champion PHC. However, this needs continued support from across the globe, as has been shown by the director-general of WHO: 'I regard universal health coverage as the single most powerful concept that public health has to offer. It is inclusive. It unifies services and delivers them in a comprehensive and integrated way, based on primary health care.'[26]

BUILD STRONG PRIMARY HEALTHCARE NETWORKS THAT CAN SUPPORT PEERS AND PROVIDE TECHNICAL ASSISTANCE AS REQUIRED

While large-scale international investments in government systems will remain important in many low-income or post-conflict countries, many international investors are now looking for innovative, non-state solutions to the development challenges of rolling out PHC. Strengthening the evidence base with rigorous evaluations of interventions to improve PHC performance can build the case for larger investments, both national and international. Networks that effectively spread the knowledge could attract considerable attention.

LOOK FOR OPPORTUNITIES FOR PRIMARY HEALTHCARE INVESTMENT

There are many opportunities already and many more on the horizon. For example, the international community is developing a more unified approach to strengthening reproductive, maternal, neonatal and child services through a new Global Financing Facility,[27] and there is an increasing interest in PHC from philanthropic donors such as the Bill & Melinda Gates Foundation.[28] Being ready for, and engaging in, these opportunities could put PHC champions in a strong place as the world moves into an era of more sustainable development.

CHAMPION INTER-SECTORIAL COLLABORATIONS AND A FOCUS ON RIGHTS

Advocates for PHC also need to bring its fundamental principles to the fore and champion improvements in the determinants of health. For instance, a partnership with the education sector is required to improve early childhood development, improve adolescent health and empower women. The agriculture sector is important to ensure food security and improved nutrition. Improved access to safe water and sanitation remains a crucially important aspect of PHC. The MDG era has also shown the importance of defending the rights of vulnerable groups, and champions of PHC must keep these arguments at the fore and build the evidence on how PHC can deliver on the opportunities arising in the post-MDG era.[29]

CHAPTER 15

Primary care research funding in the UK

. . . .

Clare Taylor and Richard Hobbs

Medical research in the UK punches well above its weight in terms of quality of research and volume (e.g. 7% of all cancer papers in 2011 originated from the UK) by investment. In 2006, the UK delivered 9% of the world's research effort for 4.5% of the world's research expenditure in a high-cost economy.[30] Indeed, the UK protected its health research budget from 2008 (although not adjusted for inflation) until 2015–2016 on the basis that such funding should attract inwards investment to the UK via commercial science funders.[31]

In terms of primary care research, the UK has several sources of funding, though mostly in open competition with all other disciplines. Broadly, primary care researchers can apply to government-funded bodies, charities or industry (pharmaceutical or medical device companies) to support their research.

The National Institute for Health Research (NIHR) in England is the research part of the National Health Service (NHS), which is funded by government through the Department of Health. With a budget of over £1 billion a year, the vision of the NIHR is 'to improve the health and wealth of the nation through research'.[32] To achieve this ambitious aim, the NIHR allocates funding to four main areas of applied health research.

First, 'infrastructure', which includes clinical research facilities and clinical research networks that support the mechanics of carrying out research and is particularly important in primary care when research studies happen across practices, coordinated by a research network. Secondly, 'faculty', which supports talented individual researchers, from trainees to senior investigators, through personal fellowships that provide salary and some research costs. The number of individuals from primary care supported by these streams is significant, and the NIHR is one of the most prominent providers of personal awards for primary care researchers; however, competition is fierce, and the overall number of fellowships awarded to primary care remains small compared with other disciplines. Thirdly, 'research programmes', which are both commissioned, when the NIHR defines the area of investigation, and researcher-led, when applicants bid competitively for a grant to fund an area of research that they feel is important and relevant to patients. Finally, 'systems', where the NIHR works to unify data input and output to streamline processes and reduce work for researchers and ensure findings from NIHR-funded projects are more accessible. All NIHR-funded research must be published open access so the results are available to policymakers, clinicians and patients globally.

Importantly for primary care research, the NIHR recognised its importance and, in 2006, set up the NIHR School for Primary Care Research. Over 90% of NHS contacts occur in the primary care setting,[33] and it is vital that research from this part of the health service is valued and funded. This is the only major research-funding stream in the UK hypothecated entirely on primary care. The school, renewed for its third 5-year term in 2015, presently comprises the nine top performing primary care research departments in England and focuses particularly on research questions relevant to primary care. Its mission is to 'increase the evidence base for primary care practice, and to increase research capacity in primary care'.[34] The school will fund £23 million of research within the nine members and £10 million on research career training posts over the next 5 years, using a competitive peer-reviewed selection process for each scheme.

The Medical Research Council (MRC) also receives government funding but from the Department for Business, Innovation and Skills via Research Councils UK rather than the Department of Health.[35] The MRC provides substantial funding for individual researchers through its fellowship programme and for research projects and programmes through its system of grants. It has also contributed to the research infrastructure through research facilities, although these are usually laboratory and hospital focused. Traditionally, the MRC has, however, funded mainly basic sciences and specialist areas rather than applied health research and, especially, not funded much primary care (although some eminent primary care researchers have been funded through the MRC, and all career stages are able to apply for its funding streams).

In addition to government, charities play a vital role in UK research funding. The Wellcome Trust is a well-known charitable foundation established in 1936 from a substantial donation in the will of Sir Henry Wellcome, a pharmaceutical entrepreneur.[36] Wellcome also funds individuals, research programmes and infrastructure, including Wellcome Trust Research Facilities. Traditionally, it has not funded primary care research significantly, although there has been some encouragement for academic general practitioners (GPs) to apply for Wellcome Trust Fellowships in recent years.[37] Other disease-specific charities include Cancer Research UK, which is responsible for around a third of the £1 billion (€1.26 billion; US$1.7 billion) a year awarded by UK medical charities to researchers,[38] and the British Heart Foundation, which offers significant funding, although this is rarely competed for successfully by primary care academics.

Industry also has a limited place in funding primary care research, and pharmaceutical companies have had a significant role in funding studies, particularly clinical trials of their products, for many years. For example, many primary care patients with atrial fibrillation (AF) take warfarin for stroke prevention. The development of novel oral anticoagulants (NOACs) could revolutionise the way patients with AF are managed. The trials to assess whether NOACs were as effective, and safe, as warfarin were sponsored by the companies that produce the products.[39-42] There is some debate about the role of industry in research. However, researchers are ethically obliged to remain independent of their funder, and without industry sponsorship, these drugs may not have been developed or trialled in such large populations. Traditionally, though, commercial research has been invested via commercial research organisations and has not sought to invest in enduring research infrastructure or focus on primary care–relevant questions.

Planning, carrying out and reporting high-quality primary care research requires a skilled workforce and, compared with hospital specialties, doctors working in primary care have been less likely to pursue a clinical academic career. The term 'academic GP' is used in the UK to describe a GP who undertakes research and/or teaching in addition to clinical duties. In a recent *BMJ* editorial, Campbell and colleagues reported that the UK has 205 senior academic GPs – just 6.5% of all clinical academics.[43] There are nearly 65 000 GPs in the UK, so academic GPs make up only 0.3% of the whole general practice workforce.[44] Yet the majority of NHS contacts occur within the primary care setting, so there is a need for funding to be focused there. Only by continuing to invest in a sustainable workforce and infrastructure will government, charities and industry ensure primary care research as a discipline has the capacity to address important research questions and improve the experience and outcomes of patients within the NHS.

CHAPTER 16

Critique of current health research funding models in Australia

. . . .

Terry Findlay and Emma Whitehead

This summary addresses how PHC research is funded in Australia, the rationale for what is prioritised and what has been achieved to date.

To build the relationship between evidence and policy development and practice in PHC, the Australian Government established the Primary Health Care Research, Evaluation and Development (PHCRED) strategy in 2000. This strategy recognised the importance of PHC, and therefore PHC research, to the health system, prioritising PHC research development so it is not left solely to compete in mainstream medical and health research funding.[45] PHCRED, which is now in its third phase, focuses on health services and systems rather than clinical research[46] and is aligned to the priority areas of the National Primary Health Care Strategy.[47]

Commissioning of research under the PHCRED strategy is undertaken by the Australian Primary Health Care Research Institute (APHCRI).[48] Commissioned research is target driven based on the current needs of policymakers, service providers and consumers. Research projects that embed stakeholders rate highly. APHCRI actively works with researchers to improve the implementation potential of research findings and develops the PHC research workforce capacity.

APHCRI's principal model of research funding is the 5-year Centre of Research Excellence programme,[49] commissioning multiple research projects in identified topic areas. Shorter-term research projects are also commissioned to reflect emerging need, with all research grants being competitive and subject to independent expert assessment.

PHCRED seeks to build research capacity through a mix of grant funding, individual and team initiatives, knowledge exchange and national and international links and collaborations. In the decade to 2013, over 800 authors[50] contributed to over 500 peer-reviewed publications supported by APHCRI. Similarly, the Primary Health Care Research and Information Service (PHCRIS), also funded through the PHCRED strategy, has provided considerable capacity-building support to researchers through information and knowledge exchange services.[51]

APHCRI's work to improve translational research, an approach endorsed by the Strategic Review of Health and Medical Research in Australia[52] and further supported by international evidence,[53,54] includes a strong history of orientating its funded research to inform policy, including a programme of knowledge translation events, the Conversations Series, with the Australian Department of Health; from 2012 to 2014, there were over 1000 attendances at Conversations Series events.[55] Furthermore, APHCRI is establishing a model to set up wide networks across broad stakeholder groups and systems to better drive the successful implementation of research into the future. This will inform government thinking on the future of Australian PHC research funding as the third phase of PHCRED concludes in 2015.[56]

CHAPTER 17

Research and primary healthcare: health systems strengthening in partner countries from a European perspective

．．．．．．．．．．．．．．．．．．．．．．．．．

*Kevin McCarthy**

Primary healthcare was recognised in the *Declaration of Alma-Ata* in 1978, with the target of 'health for all' by 2000: 'Primary health care is based on practical, scientifically sound and socially acceptable methods and technology made universally accessible … through [people's] full participation and at a cost that the community and country can afford'.[57] The World Health Organization (WHO) reaffirmed the importance of primary care in its 2008 report *Primary Care: Now More than Ever*, stressing its vision for health – physical, mental and social well-being, essential if health for all is to become a reality. The report states: 'There is a huge research agenda with enormous potential to acceler-ate the PHC [primary healthcare] reforms that requires more concerted attention … Yet, currently, the share of health expenses devoted to determining what works best – to health services research – is less that [sic] 0.1% of health expenditure in the United States … It is time for health leaders to understand the value of investment in this area'.[58]

The Sixty-Second World Health Assembly, in its 'WHA62.12: primary health care, including health system strengthening' resolution,[59] set out the principles of effective health systems, including a rights approach with inclusive leadership, and stated that health systems must include the health-in-all approach, relating health services to the sources of the main risks. Health systems must also deliver people-centred services that respond to needs at the level of care required for the principle of universal coverage. The resolution also made reference to improving access to appropriate medicines, health products and technologies, all of which are required to support primary healthcare,

---

* The information and views set out in this chapter are those of the author and do not necessarily reflect the official opinion of the European Union. Neither the European Union institutions and bodies nor any person acting on their behalf may be held responsible for the use which may be made of the information contained therein.

and to develop and strengthen health information and surveillance systems relating to primary healthcare in order to facilitate evidence-based policies and programmes and their evaluation.

In the 2004 WHO *World Report on Knowledge for Better Health*,[60] it was concluded that more investment is needed for a new innovative approach to research on health systems, that such health systems must be managed more effectively and that a stronger emphasis should be placed on translating knowledge into action to improve public health by bridging the gap between what is known and what is actually being done. The WHO *World Health Report 2013: Research for Universal Health Coverage*[61] states that universal health coverage requires a strong, efficient, well-run health system; access to essential medicines and technologies; and sufficient, motivated health workers – the challenge for most countries however, is how to expand health services to meet growing needs with limited resources. The report argues that universal health coverage – with full access to high-quality services for prevention, treatment and financial risk protection – cannot be achieved without the evidence provided by scientific research. Such research, able to address issues to improve human health, well-being and development, needs to follow a participatory approach with commitment to strengthening the appropriate capacity to make use of the research outcomes.

The discussion and, currently, the negotiations around the post-2015 agenda and the development of the Sustainable Development Goals over the last 24 months have seen the importance of research and innovation key to implementing the goals and targets that will be adopted by the United Nations in September 2015. At the same time, the Ebola outbreak has clearly illustrated the need to invest if health systems and health services are to prove resilient to such outbreaks. As Margaret Chan stated: 'As we have learned, Ebola is an unforgiving virus that can take advantage of any mistakes and exploit every opportunity to resist control.

'Weak health systems created multiple opportunities. In some areas, all forms of essential care, whether for malaria treatment or safe childbirth, have ceased to function'.[62]

SCIENCE, TECHNOLOGY AND INNOVATION

It is clear that science, technology and innovation (STI) are necessary for development. Science and technology, knowledge sharing and capacity and innovation play a vital game-changing role in empowering developing countries' economies and societies to lift them out of poverty. They are essential drivers and enablers for eradicating poverty and the achievement of the Millennium Development Goals (MDGs), as well as playing a vital role where the three pillars of sustainable development – economic, social and environmental – are concerned, facilitating efforts to address global challenges.

At the same time, useful, meaningful research, reaching those who need it, is required. Where and how – with partner countries, of course – can research bring the best benefits and gains? What kind of research are we talking about? Is it applied, operational, intervention, implementation, action-oriented or results/outcome research.

What is meant by these terms? In the final analysis, it is important to understand what works best and how, and in which local, social and economic development contexts.

EUROPEAN UNION DEVELOPMENT POLICY

The Directorate-General for International Cooperation and Development's work (EuropeAid) is carried out with the ultimate aim of reducing poverty in the world; ensuring sustainable development; and promoting democracy, peace and security. As well as designing policies to achieve these objectives, EuropeAid is responsible for implementing the European Union's (EU) external aid instruments, coordinating the actions of the EU institutions, the EU member states and other EU actors around the union's core values, objectives and common priorities.

The EU pursues a rights-based approach to health supporting 'health-in-all policies', including universal access to quality health services based on the values that EU health systems are built on. This ensures that the underlying determinants of health are addressed beyond the health sector, such as gender equality, water and sanitation, education, food and nutrition security, decent work and social protection, environmental factors and security. Strengthening all areas of a health system – with primary healthcare being a key part – and including the availability of qualified health workers, the provision of affordable medicines and adequate financing of the sector, is key to moving towards quality health services that are accessible and affordable for all.

The 2010 *Council Conclusions on the EU Role in Global Health*[63] stipulated that EU support to health 'shall ensure that the main components of health systems – health workforce, access to medicines, infrastructure and logistics, financing and management – are effective enough to deliver universal coverage of basic quality care, through a holistic and rights based approach'.

EUROPEAN UNION DEVELOPMENT POLICY AND HEALTH RESEARCH

Development cooperation and aid, and STI cannot separately take us forward. There has to be cooperation between the two – and, indeed, with other policies with important external relations effects: trade, internal market etc. At the same time, knowledge cannot simply be 'transferred' to partner countries nor can their science priorities be dictated. They need to be empowered to establish their own research policies and be supported with appropriate capacity building to carry them out.

Identifying an evidence basis to examine policy options means better linkages between research and policymaking. This depends on finding points of exchange between policy and research community that go beyond the 'outcome' or 'product' stages of each of their processes, focusing on research results/outcomes that are syntheses of a broad spectrum of knowledge, rather than an individual study's findings. Above all, research is needed in health systems to ensure affordable, sustainable benefits to those who most need them by optimising the delivery of corresponding health services. The *Council Conclusions on the 2010 Communication on the EU Role in Global*

Health[64] called on the EU and its member states to promote effective and fair financing of research that benefits the health of all. This is key to the approach EuropeAid takes in the health sector.

In the European Commission, EuropeAid does not have a mandate per se to support health research for development; rather, the EU Framework Programmes for Research are best placed to cover development policy needs. Nevertheless, some EuropeAid actions do support pertinent research and capacity building but primary healthcare is not explicitly targeted. EuropeAid actions include projects that implement elements of 'The global strategy and plan of action on public health, innovation and intellectual property',[65] thanks to the European Parliament's initiatives on the issue of access to medicines. Some €38 million has been provided in support for capacity building, local production and transfer of technology, and improved community access to health interventions when primary healthcare is concerned. The latter example provides €3 million to promote research for improved community access to health interventions in Africa (2010–2015).[66] The relevance and urgency for establishing information and practices that provide evidence for effectively scaling up the role of communities in the delivery of primary healthcare in sub-Saharan Africa, integrated within national health systems, remain high. Project work takes place in Burkina Faso, Malawi, Nigeria and Uganda. This is an example of EuropeAid being in a position to initiate support combining both research into policy and health systems / primary healthcare objectives.

Regarding the strengthening of public health institutes with the overall objective of contributing to the protection and promotion of population's health through the provision of policy analysis and policy advice, EuropeAid under the Development Cooperation Instrument 'Investing in People' currently supports eight public health institute projects. Such institutes are a key component of the development and strengthening of coherent and efficient health systems. The support aims at reinvigorating and developing institutes most often lacking sufficient resources to fulfil a significant role in the health sector. Some €22.8 million has been allocated to eight country public health institute projects: Bangladesh, Burundi, Haiti, Kenya, Laos, Morocco, Myanmar and Uganda.[67]

EUROPEAN UNION FRAMEWORK PROGRAMMES FOR RESEARCH

The main instrument for implementing the EU's research policy is The EU Framework Programme for Research and Innovation,[68] implemented by the Director-General for Research and Innovation. The EU has been financing research on the basis of multiannual framework programmes since 1984. The EU's current international cooperation strategy on research and innovation underlines cooperation with developing countries as a distinct objective. The 2012 European Commission communication on *Enhancing and Focusing EU International Cooperation in Research and Innovation: A Strategic Approach*[69] identifies developing countries as a group under Horizon 2020. The emphasis is to be on complementing the EU's external policies and instruments by building partnerships – in particular, bi-regional partnerships – to contribute to the sustainable development of these regions and address challenges such as the green economy, climate action, improved agriculture, food security and health. Furthermore, this includes 'supporting the Millennium Development Goals – and their possible successors – strengthening demand-led research and innovation for development, and delivery of the outcome of the Rio+20 conference, e.g. through the transfer of climate technologies'.[69]

HORIZON 2020 AND HEALTH RESEARCH

One of Horizon 2020's objectives is to contribute to finding solutions to societal challenges in line with the EU's international commitments – development policy included – while contributing to the sustainable development of developing countries. Societal Challenge 1, entitled 'Health, Demographic Change and Wellbeing', under Horizon 2020 aims to invest in better health for all. It aims to keep older people active and independent for longer and supports the development of new, safer and more effective interventions. Research and innovation also aims to contribute to the sustainability of health and care systems, working together across borders, sharing knowledge and resources and improving the health and care system together.[70] Horizon 2020 also supports the European and Developing Countries Clinical Trials Partnership.[71]

Regarding global health research, currently, the European Commission is the third largest contributor in the world, after the National Institutes of Health and the Bill & Melinda Gates Foundation. The significance of this priority has recently been demonstrated in the response to the Ebola crisis. Here, the European Commission rapidly mobilised nearly €250 million within 6 months specifically for emergency research on the disease. To understand the contribution of EU-funded research and development on poverty-related and neglected diseases to universal health coverage, and the improvement of the health situation in low- and middle-income countries, a study tender was launched by the European Commission in October 2015.[72]

PAST EUROPEAN UNION FRAMEWORK PROGRAMMES FOR RESEARCH

Under the Seventh Framework Programme for Research and Innovation (FP7), the European Commission committed a total of €804.7 million to global health research, including €460.7 million to the three major poverty-related diseases HIV/AIDS, tuberculosis (TB) and malaria; €168.6 million to neglected infectious diseases related to poverty; and €276.1 million to maternal reproductive and child health.

The 'health' theme of the specific programme on 'Cooperation' under FP7[73] provided a mandate for international cooperation in the context of the MDGs. Priority areas, formulated by bi-regional dialogues in non-EU countries, regions and international fora and adapted to local needs or with the aid of partnerships, included health policy research, health systems and healthcare service research, maternal and child health, reproductive health, control and surveillance of neglected communicable diseases and emerging unforeseen policy needs in the regions concerned.

The focus of research relating to international public health and health systems was of direct relevance to the international dimension of the public health policy of the EU by contributing to health protection, prevention and promotion, while, at the same time, generating new knowledge relevant to health, social, environmental and economic issues. Taking cross-sectorial and multidisciplinary approaches, this research[74] contributed to initiatives such as the MDGs, the Ministerial Declarations on global health research[75] and the EU Policy Coherence for Development framework, with particular emphasis on attaining the health MDGs, including child, maternal and reproductive health. Project examples include Consortium for Health Policy and Systems Analysis in Africa (CHEPSAA),[76] EquitAble[77] and Human Resources for Primary Health Care in Africa (HURAPRIM).[78] HURAPRIM focused on human resources for primary healthcare in Africa, while CHEPSAA's aim was to extend sustainable African capacity to produce and use high-quality health policy and systems research, by harnessing synergies among a consortium of African and European universities with relevant expertise. EquitAble was about enabling universal and equitable access to healthcare for vulnerable people in resource poor settings in Africa.

Under the Sixth Framework Programme (FP6; 2002–2006), as part of international cooperation activities (INCO), some €34 million was provided to support 20 projects on health financing, access to healthcare, quality management, health migration and reproductive health.[79] A comprehensive review, covering 43 Fifth Framework Programme and FP6 health systems research projects, confirmed the significant impact and contribution to building solid north–south partnerships.[80]

CONCLUSION

It is clear that a robust primary healthcare system is key to providing healthcare in low-income countries – indeed, the same can be said for high-income countries. To make the most efficient use of limited resources, both research and healthcare communities must collaborate to ensure a participatory approach to develop pertinent, targeted primary healthcare research. Then, to ensure the take-up of research outcomes in practice and to continue developing a strong evidence-based approach in systems and policies, this collaboration/cooperation must continue and flourish. The international community can play a key role in developing infrastructures, building capacity, encouraging networks and opportunities to facilitate this.

SECTION III REFERENCES

1. Commission for Health Research and Development. *Health Research: The Essential Link to Equity in Development.* New York, NY: Oxford University Press, 1990.
2. Sridhar D. Who Sets the global health research agenda? The challenge of multi-bi financing. *PLoS Medicine* **9**(9): e1001312.
3. McCoy D, Sanders D, Baum F et al. Pushing the international health research agenda towards equity and effectiveness. *Lancet* 2004; **364**(9445): 1630–1.
4. Gonzalez-Block MA. Health policy and systems research agendas in developing countries. *Health Research Policy and Systems* 2004; **2**(1): 6.
5. Aoun S, Pennebaker D, Pascal R. To what extent is health and medical research funding associated with the burden of disease in Australia? *Australian and New Zealand Journal of Public Health* 2004; **28**(1): 80–6.
6. Kingdon D. Health research funding: mental health research continues to be underfunded. *BMJ* 2006; **332**(7556): 1510.
7. Gillum LA, Gouveia C, Dorsey ER et al. NIH disease funding levels and burden of disease. *PLoS One* 2011; **6**(2): e16837.
8. Bird P, Omar M, Doku V et al.; MHaPP Research Programme Consortium. Increasing the priority of mental health in Africa: findings from qualitative research in Ghana, South Africa, Uganda and Zambia. *Health Policy and Planning* 2011; **26**(5): 357–65.
9. Sheikh K, George A, Gilson L. People-centred science: strengthening the practice of health policy and systems research. *Health Research Policy and Systems* 2014; **12**: 19.
10. Svoronos T, Macauley RJ, Kruk ME. Can the health system deliver? Determinants of rural Liberians' confidence in health care. *Health Policy and Planning* 2014; **30**(7): 823–9.
11. O'Hare B. Weak health systems and Ebola. *Lancet Global Health* 2015; **3**(2): e71–2.
12. Peoples Health Movement (PHM). *PHM Position Paper: Ebola Epidemic Exposes the Pathology of the Global Economic and Political System.* Peoples Health Movement, n.d. Available at: http://www.phmovement.org/sites/www.phmovement.org/files/phm_ebola_23_09_2014final_0.pdf (accessed 26 March 2015).
13. Republic of Liberia. *Millennium Development Goals 2010 Report: Progress, Prospects and Challenges towards Achieving the MDGs.* Monrovia: Ministry of Planning and Economic Affairs, 2010. Available from http://www.lr.undp.org/content/dam/liberia/docs/docs/MDG%20Report%20Liberia%202010.pdf (accessed 26 March 2015).
14. London L, Naledi T, Petros S. Health research in the Western Cape Province, South Africa: lessons and challenges. *African Journal of Primary Health Care & Family Medicine* 2014; **6**(1): E1–7.
15. Bradshaw D, Groenewald P, Laubscher R et al. Initial burden of disease estimates for South Africa, 2000. *South African Medical Journal* 2003; **93**(9): 682–8.
16. de Mello Vianna CD, Caetano R, Ortega JA et al. Flows of financial resources for health research and development in Brazil, 2000–2002. *Bulletin of the World Health Organization* 2007; **85**(2): 124–30.
17. Ranson MK, Bennett SC. Priority setting and health policy and systems research. *Health Research Policy and Systems* 2009; **7**: 27.
18. Ijsselmuiden C, Jacobs M. Health research for development: making health research work … for everyone. *Scandinavian Journal of Public Health* 2005; **33**(5): 329–33.
19. United Nations General Assembly. *International Covenant on Economic, Social and Cultural Rights.* Adopted and opened for signature, ratification and accession by General Assembly resolution 2200A (XXI) of 16 December 1966. Entered into force 3 January 1976, in accordance

with article 27. United Nations Headquarters, New York. Available at: http://www.ohchr.org/EN/ProfessionalInterest/Pages/CESCR.aspx (accessed 28 November 2015).

20. Moon S, Omole O. *Development Assistance for Health: Critiques and Proposals for Change.* Working Group on Financing: Paper 1. London: Chatham House, 2013. Available at: https://www.chathamhouse.org/sites/files/chathamhouse/public/Research/Global%20Health/0413_devtassistancehealth.pdf (accessed 27 November 2015).

21. Graves C, Haakenstad A, Dieleman JL. Tracking development assistance for health to fragile states: 2005–2011. *Globalization and Health* 2015; **11**: 12.

22. United Nations (UN) Department of Economic and Social Affairs Division for Sustainable Development. *Open Working Group Proposal for Sustainable Development Goals.* New York, NY: UN Department of Economic and Social Affairs Division for Sustainable Development, n.d. Available at: https://sustainabledevelopment.un.org/owg.html (accessed 2 February 2016).

23. World Health Organization (WHO). *The World Health Report 2008: Primary Health Care; Now More than Ever.* Geneva: WHO, 2008. Available at: http://www.who.int/whr/2008/whr08_en.pdf (accessed 24 November 2015).

24. Maeseneer JD, van Weel C, Egilman D et al. Funding for primary health care in developing countries: money from disease specific projects could be used to strengthen primary care. *BMJ* 2008; **336**(7643): 518–19.

25. Measurement and Accountability for Results in Health: A Common Agenda for the post-2015 era (MA4Health). Roadmap. Available at: http://ma4health.hsaccess.org/roadmap (accessed 12 April 2015).

26. Chan M. Universal health coverage. Available from http://www.who.int/universal_health_coverage/en/ (accessed 12 April 2015).

27. World Bank. *A Global Financing Facility in Support of Every Woman, Every Child: Concept Note.* Washington DC: World Bank, 2014. Available at: http://www.worldbank.org/content/dam/Worldbank/document/HDN/Health/ConceptNote-AGlobalFinancingFacilitySupportEveryWomanEveryChild.pdf (accessed 15 September 2015).

28. Bill & Melinda Gates Foundation. Integrated delivery: strategy overview. Available at: http://www.gatesfoundation.org/What-We-Do/Global-Development/Integrated-Delivery (accessed 12 April 2015).

29. Buse K, Hawkes S. Health in the sustainable development goals: ready for a paradigm shift? *Globalization and Health* 2015; **11**: 13.

30. Hobbs FD, Stewart PM. How should we rate research? *BMJ* 2006; **332**: 983–4.

31. HM Treasury. *Spending Round 2013.* Cm 8639. Norwich: The Stationery Office, 2013. Available at: www.gov.uk/government/uploads/system/uploads/attachment_data/file/209036/spending-round-2013-complete.pdf (accessed 27 November 2015).

32. National Institute for Health Research (NIHR). About NIHR. Available at: http://www.nihr.ac.uk/about/mission-of-the-nihr.htm (accessed 8 September 2015).

33. Royal College of General Practitioners (RCGP). *A Blueprint for Building the New Deal for General Practice in England.* London: RCGP, 2015. Available at: http://www.rcgp.org.uk/policy/rcgp-policy-areas/~/media/Files/PPF/A-Blueprint-for-building-the-new-deal-for-general-practice-in-England.ashx (accessed 27 November 2015).

34. National Institute for Health Research School for Primary Care Research. About us. Available at: http://www.spcr.nihr.ac.uk/about-us/overview (accessed 8 September 2015).

35. Medical Research Council. Spending and accountability. Available at: http://www.mrc.ac.uk/about/spending-accountability/ (accessed 8 September 2015).

36. Wellcome Trust. History of Henry Wellcome. Available at: http://www.wellcome.ac.uk/ About-us/History/index.htm (accessed 8 September 2015).

37. Wellcome Trust. Research Training Fellowships. Available at: http://www.wellcome. ac.uk/Funding/Biomedical-science/Funding-schemes/Fellowships/Clinical-fellowships/ WTD004435.htm (accessed 8 September 2015).

38. Association of Medical Research Charities (AMRC). *Charity Funded Research: AMRC Member Research Expenditure for 2012.* London: AMRC, 2013. Available at: http://www. amrc.org.uk/sites/default/files/doc_lib/AMRC%20briefing%20on%20charity%20funded%20 research%20June%202013.pdf (accessed 27 November 2015).

39. Connolly SJ, Ezekowitz MD, Yusuf S et al.; RE-LY Steering Committee and Investigators. Dabigatran versus warfarin in patients with atrial fibrillation. *New England Journal of Medicine* 2009; **361**(12): 1139–51.

40. Granger CB, Alexander JH, McMurray JJ et al.; ARISTOTLE Committees and Investigators. Apixaban versus warfarin in patients with atrial fibrillation. *New England Journal of Medicine* 2011; **365**(11): 981–92.

41. Patel MR, Mahaffey KW, Garg J et al.; ROCKET AF Investigators. Rivaroxaban versus warfarin in nonvalvular atrial fibrillation. *New England Journal of Medicine* 2011; **365**(10): 883–91.

42. Giugliano RP, Ruff CT, Braunwald E et al.; ENGAGE AF-TIMI 48 Investigators. Edoxaban versus warfarin in patients with atrial fibrillation. *New England Journal of Medicine* 2013; **369**(22): 2093–104.

43. Campbell J, Hobbs FD, Irish B et al. UK academic general practice and primary care. *BMJ* 2015; **351**: h4164.

44. Hobbs FD, Taylor CJ. Academic primary care: at a tipping point? *British Journal of General Practice* 2014; **64**(622): 214–15.

45. Anderson W. NHMRC funding for primary care research, 2000–2008. *Medical Journal of Australia* 2011; **195**(10): 583.

46. Australian Government Department of Health Standing Council on Health. *National Primary Health Care Strategic Framework.* Canberra: Department of Health, 2013. Available at: http:// www.health.gov.au/internet/main/publishing.nsf/Content/6084A04118674329CA257BF000 1A349E/$File/NPHCframe.pdf (accessed 15 September 2015)

47. Australian Government Department of Health and Ageing. *Building a 21st Century Primary Health Care System: Australia's First National Primary Health Care Strategy.* Canberra: Australian Government Department of Health and Ageing, 2010. Available at: http://www. mmgpn.org.au/media/download_gallery/COAG%202011%20Communique%20re%20 Health%20Reform.pdf (accessed 15 September 2015).

48. Australian National University Australian Primary Health Care Research Institute (APHCRI) [homepage]. Available at: http://aphcri.anu.edu.au/ (accessed 15 September 2015).

49. Australian National University APHCRI. *APHCRI Centres of Research Excellence: Evidence in Forming the Future of Australian Primary Health Care.* Canberra: APHCRI, n.d. Available at: http://aphcri.anu.edu.au/files/cre-portrait.pdf (accessed 15 September 2015).

50. APHCRI. *APHCRI: Submission to PHCRED Evaluation 2014.* Canberra: APHCRI, 2014. Available at: http://aphcri.anu.edu.au/files/submission_to_evaluation.pdf (accessed 15 September 2015).

51. Oliver-Baxter J, Brown L, Yen L et al. *Building the Primary Health Care Research Workforce in Australia.* Australian National University APHCRI and Primary Health Care Research and Information Service, 2015. Available at: http://aphcri.anu.edu.au/files/Item%205.2%20 Attachment%20APHCRI-PHCRIS%20Research%20Workforce%20Project%20Update.pdf (accessed 15 September 2015).

52. Australian Government Department of Health and Ageing. *Strategic Review of Health and Medical Research in Australia: Better Health through Research*. Final Report. Canberra: Department of Health and Ageing, 2013. Available at: http://www.mckeonreview.org.au/downloads/Strategic_Review_of_Health_and_Medical_Research_Feb_2013-Final_Report.pdf (accessed 15 September 2015).

53. Brownson RC, Allen P, Duggan K et al. Fostering more-effective public health by identifying administrative evidence-based practices: a review of the literature. *American Journal of Preventive Medicine* 2012; **43**(3): 309–19.

54. Rubenstein LV, Pugh J. Strategies for promoting organizational and practice change by advancing implementation research. *Journal of General Internal Medicine* 2006; **21**(Suppl. 2): S58–64.

55. Australian National University APHCRI. Conversations with APHCRI. Available at: http://aphcri.anu.edu.au/resources/conversations-aphcri (accessed 15 September 2015).

56. Findlay T, Whitehead E. *Primary Health Care Research in Australia: Considerations for the Future*. Canberra: Australian National University APHCRI, 2015. Available at: http://aphcri.anu.edu.au/files/Future%20of%20primary%20health%20care%20research%20in%20Australia.pdf (accessed 27 November 2015).

57. International Conference on Primary Health Care. *Declaration of Alma-Ata: International Conference on Primary Health Care, Alma-Ata, USSR, 6–12 September 1978*. Alma-Ata: World Health Organization, 1978. Available at: http://www.who.int/publications/almaata_declaration_en.pdf (accessed 24 November 2015).

58. World Health Organization (WHO). *The World Health Report 2008: Primary Health Care; Now More than Ever*. Geneva: WHO, 2008. Available at: http://www.who.int/whr/2008/whr08_en.pdf (accessed 24 November 2015).

59. WHO Sixty-Second World Health Assembly. WHA62.12: primary health care, including health system strengthening. In: *Sixty-Second World Health Assembly: Geneva, 16–22 May 2009; Resolutions and Decisions*. WHA62/2009/REC/1. Geneva: WHO, 2009. pp. 34–7. Available at: http://apps.who.int/gb/ebwha/pdf_files/WHA62-REC1/WHA62_REC1-en.pdf (accessed 27 November 2015).

60. WHO. *World Report on Knowledge for Better Health: Strengthening Health Systems*. Geneva: WHO. 2004. Available at: http://www.who.int/rpc/meetings/en/world_report_on_knowledge_for_better_health2.pdf (accessed 27 November 2015).

61. Dye C, Boerma T, Evans D et al. *The World Health Report 2013: Research for Universal Health Coverage*. Geneva: WHO, 2013. Available at: http://apps.who.int/iris/bitstream/10665/85761/2/9789240690837_eng.pdf (accessed 27 November 2015).

62. Chan M. WHO Director-General opens meeting on building resilient health systems in Ebola-affected countries. Opening remarks at a high-level meeting on building resilient health systems in Ebola-affected countries, Geneva, Switzerland, 10–11 December 2014. Available at: http://www.who.int/dg/speeches/2014/health-systems-ebola/en/ (accessed 28 November 2015).

63. Council of the European Union (EU). Point 6. In: *Council Conclusions on the EU Role in Global Health: 3011th Foreign Affairs Council Meeting, Brussels, 10 May 2010*. Brussels: EU Newsroom, 2010. p. 2. Available at: http://ec.europa.eu/health/eu_world/docs/ev_20100610_rd04_en.pdf (accessed 28 November 2015).

64. Council of the EU. Point 18. *Council Conclusions on the EU Role in Global Health: 3011th Foreign Affairs Council Meeting, Brussels, 10 May 2010*. Brussels: EU Newsroom, 2010. p. 5. Available at: http://ec.europa.eu/health/eu_world/docs/ev_20100610_rd04_en.pdf (accessed 28 November 2015).

65. WHO. The global strategy and plan of action on public health, innovation and intellectual property. Available at: http://www.who.int/phi/implementation/phi_globstat_action/en/ (accessed 28 November 2015).

66. Special Programme for Research and Training in Tropical Diseases (TDR) [homepage]. Available at: http://www.who.int/tdr/en/ (accessed 28 November 2015).

67. European Commission EuropeAid. Calls for proposals and procurement notices: Investing in People (development cooperation instrument) supporting public health institutes. Available at: https://webgate.ec.europa.eu/europeaid/online-services/index.cfm?do=publi.welcome &nbPubliList=15&orderby=upd&orderbyad=Desc&searchtype=RS&aofr=135178&user language=en (accessed 28 November 2015).

68. European Commission. Horizon 2020: what is Horizon 2020? Available at: http://ec.europa. eu/programmes/horizon2020/en/what-horizon-2020 (accessed 28 November 2015).

69. European Commission. *Communication from the Commission to the European Parliament, The Council, The European Economic and Social Committee and the Committee of the Regions: Enhancing and Focusing EU International Cooperation in Research and Innovation: A Strategic Approach.* COM(497) Final. Brussels: European Commission, 2012. Available at: http:// ec.europa.eu/research/iscp/pdf/policy/com_2012_497_communication_from_commission_ to_inst_en.pdf (accessed 28 November 2015).

70. European Commission. Horizon 2020: Health, Demographic Change and Wellbeing. Available at: http://ec.europa.eu/programmes/horizon2020/en/h2020-section/health-demographic-change-and-wellbeing (accessed 28 November 2015).

71. European and Developing Countries Clinical Trials Partnership (EDCTP) [homepage]. Available at: http://www.edctp.org/ (accessed 28 November 2015).

72. Call for tender's details: Study on poverty related and neglected diseases: evaluation of the impact of the European Union's Research Framework Programmes. No. 2015/RTD/E.3./ OP/PP-03263-2015. 6 October 2015. Available at: https://etendering.ted.europa.eu/cft/cft-document.html?docId=10623 (accessed 28 November 2015).

73. European Commission. FP7 [Seventh Framework Programme for Research and Innovation]: health. Available at: http://ec.europa.eu/research/fp7/index_en.cfm?pg=health (accessed 28 November 2015).

74. European Commission. *Public Health Research in Europe and Beyond: Project Synopses.* Reedition. Luxembourg: Publications Office of the European Union, 2011. Available at: http:// ec.europa.eu/research/health/pdf/public-health-research_en.pdf (accessed 28 November 2015).

75. Call to Action on Research for Health from the Global Ministerial Forum on Research for Health, Bamako, Mali, 17–19 November 2008. Available from www.who.int/rpc/news/ BAMAKOCALLTOACTIONFinalNov24.pdf (accessed 13 January 2016).

76. Consortium for Health Policy and Systems Analysis in Africa (CHEPSAA) [programme]. Health policy and systems resources. Available at: http://www.hpsa-africa.org/ (accessed 28 November 2015).

77. EquitAble [programme homepage]. [Coordinator: Trinity College Dublin.] Available at: http://www.equitableproject.org/ (accessed 28 November 2015).

78. Human Resources for Primary Health Care in Africa (HURAPRIM) [homepage]. Available at: http://www.huraprim.ugent.be/drupal/ (accessed 28 November 2015).

79. European Commission. *International Cooperation in FP6: Project Synopses.* EUR 22969. Luxembourg: Office for Official Publications of the European Communities, 2007. http:// ec.europa.eu/research/iscp/pdf/projects/fp6_inco_project_synopses_en.pdf

80. Van Damme W, Diesfeld H-J, Green A et al. *North South Partnership for Health Systems Research: 20 Years of Experience of European Commission Support; Report to the European Commission Summary Version.* Brussels: European Commission, 2004. Available at: https://ec.europa.eu/research/iscp/pdf/publications/n_s_partnership_health_report.pdf (accessed 28 November 2015).

SECTION IV

Primary care research organisations

Introduction

Felicity Goodyear-Smith

This section looks at the types of organisations that have developed to promote and enhance primary care research. First, there are a number of cross-nation organisations that enable researchers to meet and network, particularly at annual conferences; share ideas; and form cross-border research collaborations. Examples include the North American Primary Care Research Group (NAPCRG), the Society for Academic Primary Care (SAPC) in the UK, Primary Care and Family Medicine Education (Primafamed) Network for sub-Saharan Africa, and the the Australasian Association for Academic Primary Care (AAAPC) for Australian and New Zealand researchers.

The second part of this section documents the rise of networks of primary care practices that enable 'grassroots' practitioners to conduct meaningful research in the context in which they practice. These include primary care practice-based research networks (PBRNs) in the USA; the European General Practice Research Network (EGPRN); the Latin American Network for Research in Family Medicine (IBIMEFA), which includes the Iberian Peninsula (Spain and Portugal) as well as South America; and the International Federation of Primary Care Research Networks (IFPCRN), which was formed as a global umbrella organisation for research networks operating nationally. Chris van Weel also describes the International Implementation Research Network in Primary Care (IIRNPC), which aims to support international collaboration between researchers and other stakeholders.

Cross-nation organisations

CHAPTER 18

North American Primary Care Research Group

William Phillips

The North American Primary Care Research Group (NAPCRG) is the world's largest organisation devoted to research in family medicine, primary care and related fields, including epidemiology, behavioural sciences and health services research. NAPCRG (pronounced 'nap-crag') provides a forum for presenting new knowledge to guide improvement, redesign and transformation of primary care.

Its mission statement declares: 'NAPCRG is a volunteer association of members committed to producing and disseminating new knowledge from all disciplines relevant to primary care. NACPRG has bi-national governance (US-Canada) and international research vision and outreach. NAPCRG's Annual Meeting is the premier international forum for presenting new knowledge in primary care and advances in research methodology. NAPCRG is committed to a nurturing, informative and inspiring environment for all members.'

Founded in 1972 by Dr Maurice Wood and 50 researchers from the USA and Canada, NAPCRG was organised as a bi-national, interdisciplinary, generalist organisation. Incorporated in 1975 in Virginia as a 501(c)3 non-profit corporation, executive services were initially provided by the Medical College of Virginia in Richmond, Virginia, and, since 1995, by the Society of Teachers of Family Medicine (STFM) in Leawood, Kansas.

The governance structure reflects NAPCRG's commitment to inclusion, with representatives from the College of Family Physicians of Canada Section of Researchers,

American Board of Family Medicine (ABFM), STFM, community-based clinicians, international members, students, residents and research fellows.

Annual meetings traditionally alternate between locations in the USA and Canada, drawing members from every continent. NAPCRG and its members have made foundational contributions to primary care research, including: building capacity for primary care science; developing practice-based research networks; integration of mental health into primary care; establishing diagnostic and procedure coding; community-based participatory research; quantitative, qualitative and mixed methods research; engaging patients and communities in research; focusing on patient-centred care; addressing health in aboriginal and First Nations communities; and studies of multi-morbidity.

NAPCRG has led in developing practice-based research networks of regional, national and international scope. In 1979, it started the Ambulatory Sentinel Practice Network with support from the Rockefeller and Kellogg Foundations. Since 2012, NAPCRG has hosted the Practice-Based Research Networks Conference in Bethesda, Maryland, with support from the Agency for Healthcare Research and Quality.

Member activity is organised by special interest groups, currently including groups on cancer, community-oriented primary care, complexity science, generalism, health equity, international health literacy, medical home, mental health problems, multi-morbidity, respiratory infection, obstetrics, participatory research, patient and public involvement and engagement in primary care research, pharmacotherapy, primary care genomics, refugee and immigrant healthcare, and women in research.

NAPCRG advocates for primary care research, funding and training through work with the CFPC and membership in the Council of Academic Family Medicine, the 'family of family medicine organisations', in the USA.

The Maurice Wood Award for Lifetime Contribution to Primary Care Research is NAPCRG's highest honour, conferred every year since 1995. To nurture new investigators, the organisation offers awards to students, residents, fellows and practitioners.

Along with these organisations, NAPCRG sponsors the *Annals of Family Medicine* journal.

CHAPTER 19

Society for Academic Primary Care

· · · · · · · · · · · · · · · · · · · ·

Joanne Reeve

The Society for Academic Primary Care (SAPC) is the primary organisation championing academic primary care (APC) in the UK. The SAPC aims to provide a clear voice and a strong presence for APC in the complex and ever-changing primary care environment. It offers a point of reference and contact for those seeking academic solutions to the problems they face in the provision and study of primary care. The SAPC also provides career support to professionals seeking to develop excellence in the provision of primary care and the advancement of APC.

A detailed history of the SAPC has recently been published.[1] In brief, APC in the UK originated in the educational arm of our discipline. The first UK-funded undergraduate academic general practice (AGP) post was established in Edinburgh in 1948. With the foundation of the Royal College of General Practitioners (RCGP) in 1952 came the goal to establish a department of general practice in every medical school. The visionary work of key individuals led to the growth of AGP departments with independent chairs throughout the UK. The first AGP scientific meeting was held in 1972 in Cardiff, at which the Association of University Teachers of General Practice (AUTGP) was established. As the maturing discipline expanded its capacity for both education and research, emerging departments welcomed colleagues from multiple disciplines. The AUTGP became the Association of University Departments of General Practice, and – in 2000 – the Society for Academic Primary Care.

The SAPC today maintains its firm base within university academic departments, delivering primary care teaching and research. Its diverse membership reflects the range of professional disciplines working with and within primary care; about half of the society's members have a clinical background.[2] Reflecting the growing diversity and complexity of UK primary care, the SAPC also works with an expanding range of colleagues and organisations to support primary care improvement – including the RCGP, national Clinical Research and Academic Health Science Networks, research funders including the National Institute for Health Research, as well as international partners including the Australasian Association for Academic Primary Care / Primary Health Care Research and Information Service and NAPCRG.

The SAPC's work focuses on its three key goals:

1. to champion a vision of advancing primary care through education and research
2. to build and support a vibrant APC workforce
3. to create and sustain impact through collaborative action – activities include hosting regional and national meetings; career support for early career academics, primary healthcare scientists and academic general practitioners through providing a range of 'getting in' and 'getting on' resources; as well as outreach work with external organisations.

This work is led by the SAPC Executive, currently made up of nine elected and six co-opted members – including the chairs of the Heads of Departments and Heads of Teaching groups.[3]

CHAPTER 20 ˙

Primafamed

. . . .

Jan De Maeseneer

In 1997, at a meeting of the eight departments of family medicine and primary care in South Africa and the four Flemish departments of family medicine, *The Durban Declaration* was formulated, which outlined inter-university cooperation in the field of postgraduate training of family physicians in South Africa (www.safpj.co.za/index. php/safpj/article/view/2272). From 2003 onwards, with sponsorship from the Belgian government via the VLIR-UOS programme (www.vliruos.be), regular meetings were held that had a combined focus on training and improvement of service delivery on the one hand, and development of research on the other.

In 2006, departments of family medicine in Tanzania, Kenya, the Democratic Republic of Congo, Rwanda and Uganda joined the network, and, in 2008, the African Primary Care and Family Medicine Education (Primafamed) Network officially started, supported by the African, Caribbean and Pacific Group of States – European Union (ACP-EU) Cooperation Program in Higher Education (Edulink). This network developed a strategy to strengthen academic departments of family medicine, including the initiation of collaborative research projects. In this period, the network also extended to include Sudan, Ghana and Nigeria. A further development in 2008 was the creation of the *African Journal of Primary Health Care & Family Medicine* (www.phcfm. org), which created a platform to publish the first research output, in both English and French, from family medicine in Africa. The journal has been very successful and has recently been listed in MEDLINE and become financially self-sustaining as an open access web-based journal.

From 2009 onwards, the 'twinning project' developed. In this project, each of the departments of family medicine in South Africa 'twinned' with another country to support them in developing training of family physicians, even if that country did not yet have a medical school. In some of these twinning relationships, there was a need for development of research projects. Initially, research focused on exploring the definition and principles of family medicine in sub-Saharan Africa.[4] An international Delphi consensus study revealed that the core values and characteristics of family medicine, such as being holistic, longitudinal, comprehensive and family and community oriented, were recognised as relevant, with differences from more developed settings in terms of emphasis, organisational principles and scope of practice.[4] Several key organisational principles, such as home visiting and first contact care, were seen differently from family medicine in developed countries. Various research projects underpinned the creation of a 'Statement of consensus of family medicine in Africa' that was agreed to in a participative process at the 2nd Africa Regional World Organization of Family Doctors (WONCA) Conference.[5] This consensus stated clearly that 'research much be included in all graduate programmes'.

In the declaration at the end of the Primafamed workshop at Victoria Falls, Zimbabwe (2012), 'Scaling-up family medicine and primary health care in Africa: statement of the Primafamed Network', there was a paragraph clearly related to research:

> The participants stress that appropriate research in family medicine and primary health care in Africa is essential, in order to substantially enlarge the evidence base for the issues highlighted in this statement. This should be facilitated by the provision of specific funding by governments and non-governmental organisations (NGOs), by building the research capacity in academic departments of the family medicine and primary health care, and by developing an African Family Medicine and Primary Health Care Research Network to support researchers and promote cross-country collaboration.[6]

An example of such a project that grew out of this kind of cooperation is Human Resources for Primary Health Care in Africa (HURAPRIM),[7] a European Union–funded international research project aimed at assessing and developing interventions and policies to address the personnel crisis in the health sector, especially in Africa. The project brings together six African partners from different parts of the continent and three experienced European universities.

The 6th Primafamed workshop in Pretoria, South Africa (2014), focused on 'capacity building and priorities in primary care research'.[8] The participants concluded that there was an urgent need to:

- Create opportunities for advanced research training through doctoral degree programmes.
- Provide courses or retreats on scientific writing skills for proposals, grants, reports and publications.
- Provide courses on relevant methodologies for primary care researchers.

In response to these conclusions, the 2015 Primafamed workshop in Accra, Ghana, offered participants two full-day workshops to improve their scientific writing and research skills. The Primafamed Network, apart from its focus on capacity building in the field of family medicine training, has increasingly invested in capacity building for research in family medicine and primary healthcare in Africa.[9] This will also remain an important goal for the future development of the Primafamed Network.

CHAPTER 21

Australasian Association of Academic Primary Care

. . . .

Nick Zwar

The Australasian Association of Academic Primary Care (AAAPC) was founded in 1983 as the Australian Association for Academic General Practice (AAAGP) with 44 inaugural members under the leadership of its first president, Professor Neil Carson. The original aims of the organisation were to advance the discipline of AGP through the promotion of scholarship and innovation in research and medical education, and to represent the university departments of general practice in which the majority of senior researchers were based.

The AAAGP helped to put academics from departments around Australia in touch with each other, and this was enhanced from 1986 on with the publication of a regular newsletter. The AAAGP also developed a role in advocacy to promote general practice–based education and research. The first example was a submission to the Commonwealth Board of Inquiry into Medical Education and Medical Research in 1988. A key objective was to develop capacity in AGP research and education, and, in 1990, the AAAGP supported the publication of the first review of AGP in Australian medical schools. This advocacy work has continued since. More recent examples are a submission to the McKeon Review of Health and Medical Research and the Horvath Review of Medicare Locals.

Through the 1990s, the AAAGP worked in collaboration with the Royal Australian College of General Practitioners to promote academic sessions at the college's Annual Scientific Meetings. With the establishment of PHCRIS and the advent of annual Primary Health Care Research Conferences, the AAAGP established a close working relationship with PHCRIS, focused around the annual conference. This involves input into the conference-organising committee, association members reviewing abstracts, the AAAGP (now AAAPC) Most Distinguished Paper award and an AAAGP (now AAAPC) plenary session at which the most distinguished paper is presented. The value of the award was enhanced in 2013 through collaboration with the UK SAPC, whereby the award winner is subsidised to attend and present at the SAPC conference. Since

2000, the AAAGP has also provided an annual travelling fellowship that supports a member of the organisation to travel for academic exchange. In 2008, the organisation created the annual Bridges-Webb award, which recognises an AAAGP member who has made an international standard teaching and/or research contribution in the discipline.

The breadth of academic endeavour and the multidisciplinary nature of primary care were recognised by the AAAGP in 2012 with the organisation changing its name to the AAAPC. This also signalled the value the organisation placed on the growing number of non-medical members and their contribution to the academic development of primary care. After a number of years of discussion and exchange with New Zealand primary care academics, the AAAPC further expanded its scope in 2014 with the organisation becoming the Australasian Association for Academic Primary Care. The benefits were seen as cross-fertilisation of ideas, development of academic collaborations, expansion of the critical mass of primary care academics and therefore the ability of primary care academics to advocate on their own behalf, increase in the potential pool of reviewers for awards, and becoming an international organisation.

Throughout its history, the aims of the AAAPC have remained broadly consistent. These are currently framed as promoting and developing the discipline of general practice and primary care through encouraging originality, questioning and the exploration of ideas within the teaching and research environment, providing a forum for the exchange of information and ideas, encouraging shared academic activities, fostering and supporting career development in AGP and APC, and supporting the continuing development of AGP and APC.

Primary care research networks

Introduction

....

Andrew Bazemore

Most healthcare, addressing the majority of the problems facing its population, is delivered outside of large academic hospitals, in which the vast majority of research occurs.[10,11] Not unlike population health–minded collaborators in public and community health fields, primary care researchers face a nearly boundless array of research possibility and proportionally small research funding and training resources relative to traditional biomedical research enterprises.[12-14]

And yet, because of its broad mandate, history of engagement and delivery platform embedded in the heart of neighbourhoods, primary care research is uniquely positioned to escape the microcosmic reductionism of these same traditional enterprises and inform 'Communities of Solution' that improve population health.[15] Networks of primary care practices conducting meaningful research continue to grow globally; for example, while a handful of networks could be documented in all of North America in the early 1990s, a federal research agency in the USA listed over 130 practice-based research networks (PBRNs) in 2011, encompassing nearly 13 000 practices that cared for over 47 million people.[16] These networks are at the vanguard of community engaged and participatory research, and increasingly demonstrate their role as innovators in the interdisciplinary evaluation of how social determinants can be effectively addressed in primary care.[17,18]

CHAPTER 22

Primary care practice-based research networks

....

Rebecca Roper

Primary care practice-based research networks (PBRNs) are groups of primary care clinicians and practices working together to answer community-based healthcare questions and translate research findings into practice. They comprise groups of clinicians, diversified members of clinical teams, adept practice facilitators, informed and engaged patients, and skilled researchers. Together, they engage in an ongoing dialogue to answer community-based healthcare questions, seek and share practical solutions, translate evidence-based findings into practice and assist practitioners and practices to comply efficiently with health service transformations, such as becoming patient-centred medical homes or using electronic health records. PBRNs, in part with funding from the Agency for Healthcare Research and Quality (AHRQ), have been successful innovators of practice improvement strategies – practice facilitation, team-based care, meaningful patient engagement in health research and healthcare delivery, strategies for using health information technology – that are now considered to be essential elements of high-quality primary care. Informative project profiles describing the organisation, technical expertise and impact of PBRNs as distinctive entities and coalitions are available.[19] The AHRQ has also funded an easy-to-follow guide for new and evolving PBRNs.[20]

The AHRQ maintains a registry of PBRNs, and there are currently 174 registered PBRNs whose 153 736 clinicians serve more than 86 million patients – a 15-fold increase from the dozen PBRN registrants in 1999. The AHRQ-supported PBRN registration website[21] features informative resources and tools for would-be and evolving PBRNs. Multidimensional growth occurs as PBRNs assess and redefine their relevance. On an annual basis, each PBRN purposefully reconsiders its configuration, collaborative partnerships, mission statement, workforce, membership and business model in response to changes such as the increasing dominance of healthcare system-owned primary care practices, as well as the quest for meaningful solutions to the real-world challenges of clinicians and clinical teams.

The 'PBRN' designation has become a recognised brand for producing high-quality primary care research findings and implementation guidance – as exemplified by the fact that 85% of participants in PBRN-sponsored educational webinars[22] were not affiliated with a PBRN. National grant funders, such as the AHRQ, the National Institutes of Health Clinical and Translational Scientific Awards, the Patient-Centered Outcome Research Institute and the Centers for Medicare and Medicaid Services have recognised their value in numerous funding awards to PBRNs. In addition, established PBRNs – for example, Oregon practice-based research network (ORPRN) and Oklahoma practice-based research network (OPRN) – have made significant contributions to public health through their work for state epidemiology offices and state Medicaid offices. By applying their expertise in practice improvement, PBRNs are able to market their skills to enable others, often the underserved, to benefit from improved access to healthcare and hope for a higher quality of life.

PBRNs are leveraging their infrastructure to further serve their members by integrating programs that provide their practitioners with medical education credits and the quality improvement training required by relevant medical boards.

Several aspects of primary care are changing rapidly, including financing, electronic record keeping and integration of healthcare systems. The PBRNs are poised to inform how emerging, integrated electronic data repositories can be used to develop robust standardised primary care datasets. As PBRNs reconfigure their sustainability models, they will seek to optimise their opportunities to market their practice improvement expertise without marginalising their practice-based research activities. The camaraderie and commitment displayed among this community indicate its willingness to pursue a path of constructive evolution that assures the continuing relevance of PBRNs in an ever-changing environment.

CHAPTER 23

International Federation of Primary Care Research Network

· ·

Christos Lionis

The International Federation of Primary Care Research Networks (IFPCRN) was formed under the WONCA Task Force on Research at the May 2001 meeting in Durban, South Africa. Nineteen individuals from seven countries participated. Chris van Weel, on behalf of the WONCA Task Force on Research, encouraged the development of the IFPCRN and supported the list server and website for the IFPCRN (www. ifpcrn.org).

Regional representatives are involved from various countries in Africa, the Asia Pacific region, Europe, South Asia and North America. In addition, there are numerous research networks participating globally, from countries such as Brazil, Austria, Australia, Bangladesh and Belgium.

The mission of the IFPCRN is to support research for primary healthcare for the benefit of patients by:

- the mutual support of research networks
- the exchange of ideas and methodologies
- advocacy for the quality of research in primary care
- capacity building
- policy and advocacy initiatives
- doing collaborative research.

John Beasley from the USA was selected as interim chair, Helen Smith (chair of the UK Federation of Primary Care Research Network) followed, then Prof. Francisco Gómez-Clavelina from Mexico, Prof. Waris Qidwai from Pakistan, and finally, Prof. Christos Lionis from Greece. John Beasley is executive member at large and counsellor of the Steering Committee.

At a small, informal meeting of some IFPCRN members at the 2001 North

American Primary Care Research Group meeting in Halifax, some preliminary criteria for international projects were established:

- an energetic and committed principal investigator (PI) and support by clinicians in various countries
- the question to be answered is of importance and interest to local clinicians
- clear evidence of why an international approach is needed to answer the question.

The IFPCRN holds formal meetings at most WONCA conferences, including WONCA World, WONCA Europe, NAPCRG and other venues as resources permit. IFPCRN members have made numerous presentations.

Membership in the IFPCRN has developed rapidly and now includes 153 individuals and representatives of 53 networks or planned networks in 45 different countries.

The mission of the IFPCRN is in line with the recommendations of WONCA that were endorsed in the invitational conference that was held in Kingston, Ontario, Canada, in March 2003.[23]

At the WONCA Asia Pacific Regional Conference in Cebu, Philippines, in February 2011, the role of the federation in designing and implementing a regional study was discussed, and a five-step approach approved. A similar discussion was had and suggestions were raised at the 2013 WONCA World Conference in Prague.

Efforts in reconstructing and expanding the mission and functions of this network were considered after Prague. The core mission of the network was revitalised and efforts have been undertaken towards a new cycle in the life of the network. Towards that direction, a discussion about the development of practice-based rural research networks has been initiated under the support of the European Rural and Isolated Practitioners Association (EURIPA) and a consensus paper has recently been published.[24] This paper revisits the definition of practice-based research in rural family medicine, reflects on the current situation in Europe and discusses its rationale in rural family medicine. It anticipates actions in certain directions either by the EGPRN, the WONCA Working Party on Research and/or the IFPCRN. Similar policy documents need to be promoted in other regions and the IFPCRN should play a key role in that direction.

CHAPTER 24

European General Practice Research Network

....

Mehmet Ungan

The European General Practice Research Network (EGPRN) is an organisation of general practitioners (GPs) / family physicians (FPs) and other professionals involved in research in primary care in Europe. It is a major network in World Organization of Family Doctors (WONCA) Europe. There are 32 countries represented in the council, 273 individual and 33 institutional members with seven elected members on the executive board. The EGPRN office is located in the Department of Family Medicine, University of Maastricht.

In October 1971, a few academics and researchers in primary care met to develop international cooperation in Leusden, Netherlands. The European General Practice Research Workshop (EGPRW; former name) was created by those interested in research. Meetings were organised by GPs from different countries, sometimes with the help of national colleges and GP associations, when these existed. Seventy-nine regular bi-annual meetings have been organised over the last 40 years, since November 1974.

In the first 10 years, the main activity was systematic constructive criticism of research methods on research studies from individual members. Advanced statistical methodology, quantitative and qualitative research techniques also took place later. The EGPRN has been involved in a number of European studies on topics such as home visits, physical burnout and Eurobstacle (obstacles to adherence in living with type-2 diabetes).

With the amalgamation in 1995 of the European Society of General Practice / Family Medicine (ESGP/FM) and WONCA Region Europe, the EGPRN has been recognised as one of the key network organisations. A historic meeting was held in Ankara, Turkey (May 2003), at which the council decided to change the name from 'EGPRW' (Workshop) to 'EGPRN' (Network). The EGPRN raised the quality and output of its meetings, without losing its typical friendly atmosphere. The EGPRN keeps in contact with other research organisations to build research capacity in family medicine.

The EGPRN has a public website[25] including a database of past abstracts, country reports, position papers published in European journals to summarise each conference's proceedings, and the 'Research Agenda for General Practice/Family Medicine and Primary Health Care in Europe'[26] as a reference document. The EGPRN provides services to its members such as mentoring, networking with like-minded researchers, research discussions, methodology workshops and the publication of selected research abstracts in the *European Journal of General Practice*, to which members have free online access. The EGPRN is open for individual and institutional memberships, via online registration.

The meetings include oral sessions on a predetermined conference theme, as well as free-standing papers, 'one-slide / five-minutes' presentations and guided poster sessions. There are at least two keynote speakers invited by the board to each meeting to address the research on the specific conference theme. A poster prize ceremony is also one of the events for the young researchers. There are pre-conference training workshops on specific topics and/or collaborative research. There has always been a social night for dinner and dancing – a tradition that improves collaboration. EGPRN meetings are popular with both senior and junior researchers, because they facilitate easier and closer relationships. Selected meeting abstracts are published twice a year in the *European Journal of General Practice*. The EGPRN, together with national colleges and academic bodies, also organises international courses on research methodology in PHC, offering the expertise of international teaching staff.

CHAPTER 25

International Implementation Research Network in Primary Care

....

Chris van Weel

For most countries in the world, strengthening primary healthcare is a critical strategy to secure sustainable healthcare.[27] Comparison of experiences between countries is a powerful means to support system change and primary healthcare policy implementation.[28] The International Implementation Research Network in Primary Care (IIRNPC) has as its aims to support international collaboration between researchers and other stakeholders.[29] The IIRNPC was founded after the International Learning on Increasing the Value and Effectiveness of Primary Care (I LIVE PC) Conference in Washington DC in 2011, at which seven countries presented their primary healthcare experiences in health systems reform to inform US policymakers.[30]

The IIRNPC sets out to support researchers in the field of health systems and implementation research, in such a way that research can support the ability of primary healthcare to respond to the needs of individuals and communities in a broad social, economic, political and cultural context.[31] Research is a means to develop primary healthcare, by creating knowledge that informs the directions and strategies to change and improve healthcare. The IIRNPC aims to set a stage on which researchers can present their work and engage with other stakeholders in the development of primary healthcare to review the best application of that knowledge in instigating change. Through this interaction, research will empower agents of change. Research may support health systems' reform in different ways, such as in measuring performance, evaluating innovations, exploring the environment in which healthcare reform takes place and structuring the engagement of stakeholders.

The IIRNPC has defined guiding principles in primary healthcare policy implementation that shape the role of implementation research:[32]

- The top-down principle of primary healthcare development has to be translated to a bottom-up process to tailor the primary healthcare facilities towards local needs.
- In tailoring towards local circumstances, multiple stakeholders must be engaged

with healthcare professionals, policymakers, community leaders, insurers, scientists, employers and, in particular, the population that will use primary healthcare. This requires a methodology to promote meaningful engagement – above all, with those in highest need, who are often the most difficult to reach.

- There is a need to understand the prevailing health system and how it connects to the population – the priorities for change, the strengths and weakness in coping with change.

The inaugural event that triggered the founding of the IIRNPC – the I LIVE PC Conference[30] – featured the experiences of seven countries' health systems: Australia, Canada, Denmark, New Zealand, the Netherlands, England and Scotland, in addition to the USA. Although this represented a rich source of comparison, it also signalled a clear bias towards high-income countries' primary healthcare. As primary healthcare is to form the core of every health system, there is a priority to document and critically appraise all health systems around the world. The WONCA/NAPCRG toolkit[33] which provides presentation and manuscript templates makes it possible to take the first steps in this process.

An issue in the current debate on implementing primary healthcare policy is that it is presented as a one-off need of change, in which the successful introduction of a primary healthcare–based health system is presented as the end point. However, adaptation to new circumstances is a constant imperative in (primary) healthcare, as when populations and socio-economic circumstances change, health needs may change. And, with the development of new prevention and treatment, the health system's ability to respond may change. This asks for the ongoing monitoring of needs and provisions, a monitoring that falls, in particular, on primary healthcare as the sector that connects with society. The capacity to monitor and assess needs and provisions is essential to make sure that health systems stay in touch with, and ahead of, the challenges in the population – and are able to change constantly. The long-term objective of the IIRNPC is to help build a global research capacity into the operational capacity of primary healthcare to fulfil this monitoring and assess function – throughout the world.

CHAPTER 26

Latin American Network for Research in Family Medicine[*]

*Jacqueline Ponzo, Thiago Trindade, José Ramirez Aranda,
Sandro Rodrigues Batista and Sergio Minué*

The research in family medicine and primary care in Latin America is going through a time of discovery, development and consolidation. Emerging paradigms, which have implications for the world of research, offer new questions and answers to theoretical and methodological issues. Jaime Breilh[34] (Ecuador), Naomar de Almeida Filho (Brazil)[35] among many others from Brazil[36] and Argentina[37] are some contemporary examples of researchers who have contributed in recent decades to the conceptual construction of *complexity* as a paradigm in health, with a territorial and community perspective. At the same time, Latin America has not been immune to the influence of Barbara Starfield,[38] particularly in services and health systems research and their assessment through the Primary Care Assessment Tool (PCAT). Argentina, Brazil, Spain and Uruguay benefited from her direct cooperation in adapting the instrument to each country.

The practice of research in Latin America faces the usual difficulties in responding to the lack of firm policies for its development, including the allocation of resources (funding, time, and training). This was analysed in depth by the Ibero American Confederation of Family Medicine (Spanish acronym 'CIMF') at the fourth summit, held in Asunción in 2011.[39] At the same time, in contrast with this scenario of shortage, the first Ibero American Workshop on Research in Family Medicine was held in Cali (2008) (emulating the meeting in Ontario, 2003),[23] and resulting in the installation of the Latin American Network for Research in Family Medicine (IBIMEFA).[39] The assessment conducted in 2011 showed the need for further action to develop research and the network.[40] By then, WONCA-CIMF was simultaneously becoming aware of the issue,

---

[*] The Latin American Network for Research in Family Medicine includes the Iberian Peninsula (Spain and Portugal), but this text addresses the situation in Latin America: Andean Countries, Middle and Southern Cone.

and primary care research began to feature more prominently in the WONCA-CIMF summits, with academic family physicians taking the lead. In April 2014, the fifth summit had research integrated as one of its five major themes. A survey was conducted, which included 17 Latin American countries, that identified 60 active research groups (22 in the Southern Cone, 16 in Andean Countries, 11 in Mesoamerica and 11 in the Iberian Peninsula). More than half of the research reported (52.8%) focused on clinical issues and management (30.3% and 22.5%, respectively).

This stage ended with the 2nd Latin American Research in Family Medicine and Primary Care Workshop (Spanish acronym 'tiimfap2') held in Montevideo (March 2015),[40] from which the IBIMEFA was resized and reactivated based on active groups, networks and researchers. Mexico and Brazil have national networks of primary care researchers and there are experiences of north–south cooperation in projects developed within the community with teams of family and community medicine professionals (e.g. Happy Audit – South America, Center of Excellence for Cardiovascular Health in South America [CESCAS][41]); there is also south–south and intra-regional collaborative research (i.e. PCAT Ibero America Collaboration, which brings together Argentina, Bolivia, Brazil, Colombia, Ecuador, Spain, Mexico and Uruguay). The survey, conducted with more than 100 participants from tiimfap2, found that over 50% of researchers had master's or doctorate degrees.

The number and quality of reviewed and indexed journals specific to the discipline continue to grow. A meeting of editors as part of the Research Workshop was held in Montevideo, marking the beginning of interconnected work on the development of journals in each country. There are currently family and community medicine-specific journals in Argentina (*Archivos de Medicina General y Familiar*), Brazil (*Revista Brasileira de Medicina de Familia e Comunidade*), Mexico (*Revista Mexicana de Medicina Familiar*) and Venezuela (*Revista Médico de Familia*), as well as Portugal (*Revista Portuguesa de Medicina Geral e Familiar*) and Spain (*Atención Primaria, Actualización en Medicina de Familia*).

There is some tension between a vision that targets English journals with a high impact factor (IF) for the publication of Latin American primary care research, and a vision that emphasises the need for the best papers to be published in local journals and in the languages of the region, even if they do not have a high IF, as a way to enhance their development and diffusion in Ibero America. Since Montevideo, the connection between researchers and groups is growing, and many research questions can only be answered by research in family and community medicine. The Working Groups of WONCA-CIMF address the needs of young family physicians, rural practice, education and quaternary prevention, and also drive the research questions.

The websites of the IBIMEFA (www.facebook.com/ibimefa and http://ibimefa.blogspot.com/) will be developed in the next year.

SECTION IV REFERENCES

1. Howie JG, Whitfield M, editors. *Academic General Practice in the UK Medical Schools, 1948–2000: A Short History.* Edinburgh: Edinburgh University Press, 2011.

2. Calitri R, Adams A, Atherton H et al. Investigating the sustainability of careers in academic primary care: a UK survey. *BMC Family Practice* 2014; **15**(1): 205.

3. Society for Academic Primary Care [homepage]. Available at: www.sapc.ac.uk (accessed 30 November 2015).

4. Mash B, Downing R, Moosa S et al. Exploring the key principles of family medicine in sub-Saharan Africa: international Delphi consensus process. *South African Family Practice* 2008; **50**(3): 60–65.

5. Mash B, Reid S. Statement of consensus of family medicine in Africa. *African Journal of Primary Health Care & Family Medicine* 2010; **2**(1).

6. De Maeseneer J. Scaling-up family medicine and primary health care in Africa: statement of the Primafamed network, Victoria Falls, Zimbabwe. *African Journal of Primary Health Care & Family Medicine* 2013; **5**(1).

7. Human Resources for Primary Health Care in Africa (HURAPRIM) [homepage]. Available at: http://www.huraprim.ugent.be/drupal/ (accessed 28 November 2015).

8. Mash B, Essuman A, Ratansi R et al. African Primary Care Research: Current situation, priorities and capacity building. *African Journal of Primary Health Care & Family Medicine* 2014; **6**(1).

9. Goodyear-Smith F. Sub-Saharan Africa fast-tracks towards family medicine. *Family Practice* 2014; **31**(4): 371–2.

10. White KL, Williams TF, Greenberg BG. The ecology of medical care. *New England Journal of Medicine* 1961; **265**: 885–92.

11. Green LA, Fryer GE Jr, Yawn BP et al. The ecology of medical care revisited. *New England Journal of Medicine* 2001; **344**(26): 2021–5.

12. Lucan SC, Barg FK, Bazemore AW et al. Family medicine, the NIH, and the medical-research roadmap: perspectives from inside the NIH. *Family Medicine* 2009; **41**(3): 188–96.

13. Lucan SC, Phillips RL Jr, Bazemore AW. Off the roadmap? Family medicine's grant funding and committee representation at NIH. *Annals of Family Medicine* 2008; **6**(6): 534–42.

14. Lucan SC, Bazemore AW, Xierali I et al. Greater NIH investment in family medicine would help both achieve their missions. *American Family Physician* 2010; **81**(6): 704.

15. American Board of Family Medicine Young Leaders Advisory Group. Improving America's health requires community-level solutions: Folsom revisited. *American Family Physician* 2012; **86**(4): 1–2.

16. Peterson KA, Lipman PD, Lange CJ et al. Supporting better science in primary care: a description of practice-based research networks (PBRNs) in 2011. *Journal of the American Board of Family Medicine* 2012; **25**(5): 565–71.

17. Dulin MF, Tapp H, Smith HA et al. A trans-disciplinary approach to the evaluation of social determinants of health in a Hispanic population. *BMC Public Health* 2012; **12**: 769.

18. Plaut T, Landis S, Trevor J. Enhancing participatory research with the community oriented primary care model: A case study in community mobilization. *American Sociologist* 1992; **23**(4): 56–70.

19. Agency for Healthcare Research and Quality (AHRQ). PBRN profiles. Available at: http://pbrn.ahrq.gov/pbrn-profiles (accessed 29 November 2015).

20. North American Primary Care Research Group. *PBRN Research Good Practices (PRGP).* Leawood, KS: North American Primary Care Research Group, 2014. Available at: http://www.

napcrg.org/Portals/51/Documents/PBRN%20Conf%20Handouts/PRGP%202014-09-29.pdf (accessed 29 November 2015).

21. AHRQ. Practice-Based Research Networks [homepage]. Available at: http://pbrn.ahrq.gov/ (accessed 29 November 2015).

22. AHRQ. AHRQ Primary Care [YouTube channel]. Available at: https://www.youtube.com/ user/AHRQprimarycare (accessed 29 November 2015).

23. van Weel C, Rosser WW. Improving health care globally: a critical review of the necessity of family medicine research and recommendations to build research capacity. *Annals of Family Medicine* 2004; **2** (Suppl. 2): S5–16.

24. Klemens-Ketis Z, Kurpas D, Tsiligianni I et al. Is a practice-based rural research network feasible in Europe? *European Journal of General Practice* 2015; **21**(3): 203–9.

25. European General Practice Research Network [homepage]. Available at: http://www.egprn. org/ (accessed 29 November 2015).

26. Hummers-Pradier E, Beyer M, Chevallier P et al. The Research Agenda for General Practice/ Family Medicine and Primary Health Care in Europe. Part 1. Background and methodology. *Eur J Gen Pract*. 2009; **15**(4): 243–50.

27. World Health Organization. *The World Health Report 2008: Primary Health Care; Now More than Ever*. Geneva: WHO, 2008. Available at: http://www.who.int/rpc/meetings/en/ world_report_on_knowledge_for_better_health2.pdf (accessed 27 November 2015).

28. Kidd M, editor. *The Contribution of Family Medicine to Improving Health Systems: A Guidebook from the World Organization of Family Doctors*. London: Radcliffe Publishing, 2013.

29. Australian Primary Health Care Research Institute. International Implementation Research Network in Primary Care [homepage]. Available at: http://aphcri.anu.edu.au/research/ international-implementation-research-network-primary-care-iirnpc (accessed 29 November 2015).

30. Phillips RL Jr. International Learning on Increasing the Value and Effectiveness of Primary Care (I LIVE PC). *Journal of the American Board of Family Medicine* 2012; **25**(Suppl. 1): S2–5.

31. Tollman S. Community oriented primary care: origins, evolution, applications. *Social Science & Medicine* 1991; **32**(6): 633–42.

32. van Weel C, Turnbull D, Whitehead E et al. International collaboration in innovating health systems. *Annals of Family Medicine* 2015; **13**(1): 86–7.

33. WONCA Working Party on Research. Plenary panel project resource documents. Available at: http://www.globalfamilydoctor.com/groups/WorkingParties/Research/plenarypanel projectresourcedocuments.aspx (accessed 29 November 2015).

34. Breilh J. *Epidemiología Crítica: Ciencia Emancipadora e Interculturalidad* [Portuguese]. Buenos Aires: Lugar Editorial, 2003.

35. de Almeida Filho N, Lemus JD. *Epidemiología sin Números: Una Introducción Crítica a la Ciencia Epidemiológica* [Portuguese]. Washington DC: Organización Panamericana de la Salud, 1992.

36. Tarride MI. *Saúde Pública: Uma Complexidade Anunciada* [Public health complexity] [Portuguese]. Rio de Janeiro: Fiocruz, 1998.

37. Rovere M. Redes en salud: un nuevo paradigma para el abordaje de las organizaciones y la comunidad [Health Networks: a new paradigm for addressing community organizations]. Rosario: Ed. Secretary of Public Health/AMR, Institute Lazarte (reprint), 1999: 113.

38. Universidad de la República (web). Barbara Starfield: La medicina familiar está orientada a la persona, no a la enfermedad [Family medicine is aimed at the person, not the disease] (notice) 2010 (Nov 5) Spanish. Available at: www.universidad.edu.uy/prensa/renderItem/ itemId/26822 (accessed 29 November 2015).

39. World Organization of Family Doctors (WONCA) – Ibero American Confederation of Family Medicine (CIMF). *IV Cumbre Iberoamericana de Medicina Familiar* [Fourth Iberoamerican summit of family medicine]: *Carta de Asunción* [Spanish]. Asunción: WONCA-CIMF, 2011. Available at: http://buenaspracticasaps.cl/wp-content/uploads/2014/07/Carta-de-Asuncion-IV-Cumbre-Iberoamericana-de-MF-Nov-2011.pdf (accessed 29 November 2015).

40. WONCA Iberoamerica-CIMF Cumbre Iberoamericana de Medicina Familiar. *2° Taller Iberoamericano de Investigación en Medicina Familiar y Atención Primaria* [Second workshop of Iberoamerican research in family medicine and primary care] *(tiimfap2): Convocatoria* [Call]. Montevideo: WONCA Iberoamerica-CIMF CIdMFyC, 2015. Available at: www.montevideo2015wonca-cimf.org/es/Pages/JORNADASPRECONGRESO/TALLERMEDICI NAFAMILIARYATENCI%C3%93NPRIMARIA (accessed 29 November 2015).

41. Rubinstein A, Irazola V, Poggio R et al. Detection and follow-up of cardiovascular disease and risk factors in the Southern Cone of Latin America: the CESCAS I study. *BMJ Open* 2011; **1**(1): e000126.

SECTION V

National perspectives on primary care research

Introduction

....

Bob Mash and Felicity Goodyear-Smith

This final section of the book provides case histories of primary care research in 20 countries from the seven World Organization of Family Doctors (WONCA) regions of the world: Europe, Eastern Mediterranean, South Asia, Asia Pacific, Africa and the North and South Americas. The authors were asked to structure their articles by considering the history of primary care research in their country, current research activity, the gains and the challenges in developing their research capacity and the directions they foresee research heading in the future.

Four common themes emerge regarding capacity building in primary care research in both resource-rich and resource-poor nations: the development of academic departments and appointment of chairs in family medicine, resources and funding, the importance of collaboration and the diversity of research conducted. The availability of these elements is identified as facilitating the growth of primary care research in a country, whereas the lack of one or more is seen as a barrier.

DEVELOPMENT OF ACADEMIC DEPARTMENTS AND APPOINTMENT OF CHAIRS IN FAMILY MEDICINE

The growth of primary care research has largely been predicated by the development of general practice and primary care as a discipline, with the establishment of academic departments and professorial appointments in universities with a mandate to perform research. This ranges from the UK, which started this in the 1960s and now has academic general practice departments in every undergraduate medical school, to India, where a goal is for family medicine to be promoted as a distinct academic discipline. Linking research to undergraduate and postgraduate training requirements drives a baseline level of primary care research activity and creates a cohort of more established researchers. The development of research leaders at doctoral and post-doctoral levels is key.

There is a need for formal training courses that target the typical methods used in primary care research. The low levels of capability and capacity for primary care research among primary care providers are currently a limiting factor in many countries. The development of academic career pathways and linking research outputs to promotion or other incentives encourage research. The development of national journals and national family medicine or primary care conferences fosters a culture of research publication and presentation.

RESOURCES AND FUNDING

Low levels of funding for primary care research is also a limiting factor for many countries. A governmental policy commitment to universal coverage and strong primary healthcare is seen as a precursor to awareness of the importance of primary care research. A specific focus on primary care research within national funding bodies, or specific bodies set up nationally to fund and prioritise primary care research, is identified as an important driver in developing research capacity. External funding may also enable research activities, but this may mean that the research agenda is not determined by those in the recipient country.

Information feedback can facilitate primary care research. The analysis and reporting on the national state of primary care research and priorities may play an important role in influencing funding bodies at a national level.

COLLABORATION

One of the main drivers in facilitating the growth of primary care research capacity is collaboration at a variety of levels. This includes collaboration between academic departments regionally or nationally and the establishment of dedicated networks. This leads to the possibility for larger-scale multicentre studies and the consolidation of one voice about the priorities and needs. Developing networks of primary care providers or sentinel practices that can contribute to larger studies is helpful.

Collaboration also occurs across disciplines, and alliances between primary care researchers, public health researchers and behavioural scientists are strong combinations. There is also the growth of international networks, with collaboration facilitating some very large multi-country trials; for example, European Union funding supporting cross-nation research within the UK and Europe.

DIVERSITY OF RESEARCH

One of the hallmarks of primary care research is diversity with respect to type and methodology. Typical focus areas for primary care research include the following (also reflected in the typology discussed in 'The nature of primary care research' in Chapter 2):

- Clinical research on the presentation, assessment of undifferentiated problems, diagnosis and management of diseases across the burden of disease. Themes within such clinical research include whole-person medicine, patient-centredness, dealing with multi-morbidity, mental health problems and chronic conditions.

- Health services research addresses issues of access, continuity, coordination of care and comprehensiveness (health promotion, disease prevention, palliative care).
- Health systems research particularly focuses on identifying and responding to the social determinants of ill health as well as issues of gatekeeping, distributive justice and ethical / evidence-based use of resources.
- Educational research focuses on creating a primary care workforce that is fit for purpose.

As primary care research develops, it moves from descriptive small-scale studies to analytical and experimental larger-scale studies. Primary care research embraces alternative methods such as participatory action research and mixed methods that combine qualitative and quantitative approaches. There is a growing body of research on programme evaluation and the use of translational and implementation methods.

The emergence of electronic medical records and IT systems in primary care is a huge opportunity for obtaining big data and having the power to address important research questions. Further, the new field of genetics and biobanking should not be ignored by primary care researchers.

Collectively, these case histories discussed in the following chapters provide a snapshot of the state of primary care research throughout the world and highlight the challenges facing nations to obtaining an evidence base to inform primary care practice and policy.

Europe Region

CHAPTER 27

Primary care research in the UK

....

Tony Kendrick

HISTORY

One of the fundamental prerequisites for our discipline to be taken seriously in research was the appointment of professors of academic general practice in every undergraduate medical school, which was started by Edinburgh Medical School in 1963 and continued most recently by St Andrews in 2008.[1] The academic general practitioners (GPs) in these departments gathered experts in clinical topics and methodological design around them, leading to the development of multidisciplinary teams including allied health professionals, social and behavioural scientists, statisticians, health economists and data managers.[2]

National research reports were produced by leading academic GPs, which led to dedicated primary care funding initiatives in the early 2000s from the government's Medical Research Council[3] and National Health Service (NHS) Research and Development (R&D) programme,[4] including project grants and doctoral and post-doctoral fellowships.

Over the last 10 years, we have benefitted greatly from the establishment of the NHS R&D-funded National Institute for Health Research (NIHR), which provides a range of streams for all stages of the applied research process, including programme and project grants for clinical trials, cohort studies, qualitative and observational studies, health services research and research into the mechanisms of new interventions.[5]

Since 2006, the establishment of the NIHR-funded national School for Primary Care Research (SPCR), a collaboration between academic departments across England (initially five, now nine) selected for their international-level research quality, has encouraged the development of larger multicentre trials and cohort studies.[6] Scotland

and Wales also have national schools for primary care research, which means that their departments can speak with one voice and obtain support collaboratively, rather than waste effort in competing with each other.

CURRENT ACTIVITY

Multicentre trials, funded by the NIHR Health Technology Assessment programme, often costing in excess of £1 million, are directed at identifying interventions that will make a difference to patient care within 5 years of completion. Examples include the Positive Online Weight Reduction (POWER) trial of online support for self-management of obesity, led by Paul Little in Southampton,[7] and the Collaborative Care in Screen-Positive Elders with Major Depressive Disorder (CASPER-PLUS) trial of collaborative care management for older people with depression, led by Simon Gilbody in York.[8]

Analyses of routinely collected general practice data from large representative databases including the General Practice Research Database (GPRD), QResearch, and The Health Improvement Network (THIN), often include hundreds of thousands of patients and can give important insights into the current management of conditions and the needs of patients. Examples include analysis of GPRD data led by Mike Moore in Southampton – showing that the year-on-year rise in antidepressant prescribing was due to patients remaining on treatment for longer rather than any increase in the numbers of people being started on treatment, and calling for a new focus on monitoring and reviewing long-term treatment[9] – and an analysis of THIN data led by David Osborne at University College London (UCL) that showed that financial incentives in the GP Quality and Outcomes Framework led to significant improvements in the physical health screening of people with severe mental illness.[10]

Applied health research programmes, again directed at improving patient care within 5 years of completion, are funded by the NIHR up to a total of £2.5 million over 5 years, and allow teams to develop new interventions, conduct pilot and qualitative work to demonstrate their feasibility, and go on to test them in a trial. Examples include the Integrating Digital Interventions into Patient Self-Management Support (DIPSS) programme, led by Lucy Yardley, Paul Little and Mike Thomas in Southampton, on digitally supported self-management support, with hypertension and asthma work streams,[11] and the Prescribing ANtiDepressants Appropriately (PANDA) programme on identifying the indications for likely benefit from antidepressants for people with mild to moderate depression, led by Glyn Lewis at UCL.[12]

European Union (EU) funding, which must involve several countries, has facilitated the development of some very large multi-country trials. For example, the Genomics to Combat Resistance against Antibiotics for Community-Acquired Lower Respiratory Tract Infection (LRTI) in Europe (GRACE) consortium produced two of the largest trials of antibiotic use to date, both led by Paul Little: the GRACE trial of amoxicillin for lower respiratory tract infection (with 2061 patients), and the GRACE–Internet

Training for Reducing Antibiotic Use (INTRO) trial of Internet training of GPs in the use of antibiotics for acute respiratory infection (with 4264 patients).[13]

GAINS AND CHALLENGES

The greatest capability in the UK currently lies in the national collaborations between the top academic departments of general practice and primary care; in achieving more multicentre trials, cohort studies, data syntheses and programmes of mixed quantitative and qualitative research; and in training doctoral and postdoctoral research leaders of the future.

The main challenges are threats to the NHS and its currently relatively generous research funding arising from the economic recession, and a fear that underfunded and overstretched general practices will drop out of doing research.

FUTURE DIRECTIONS

The most promising opportunities for further primary care research that matter a lot to our country include the use of the Internet to support patient decision-making and access to information and support for self-management, like the POWER trial and the DIPSS programme.

New opportunities to do large-scale research are presented by the large databases of GP computerised medical records,[9,10] and EU funding for multi-country studies.[13]

Finally, the UK Biobank database of 500 000 volunteers will allow research into the genetic and developmental causes of problems, involving ongoing lifetime follow-up through GP records. For example, I am currently involved in an analysis of Biobank data on the relationship between low birth weight and the lifetime risk of depression, led by Danny Smith in Glasgow, having led previous research into this issue on the Southampton Women's Survey cohort.[14] Academic primary care research needs to extend into examining the epidemiology and causes of conditions as well as their management, and this, for me, is one of the most important future directions.

CHAPTER 28

Primary care research in Denmark

Peter Vedsted and Per Kallestrup

HISTORY

Since 1960, Danish general practice has evolved into a specialty based on a comprehensive training system and an academic discipline. The Nordic welfare model formed a basis for the full introduction of tax-financed healthcare with universal coverage, and every citizen could be listed with a general practitioner (GP). Thus, all GPs should have a contract and the number of GPs was regulated based on population size. Nationally negotiated schemes on remuneration and patient rights led to an increased focus on knowledge about the work in general practice. Therefore, in 1974, the first institute with a professor in family medicine was established. Following that, family medicine became a mandatory part of the university medical curriculum and the training of doctors. In 1994, family medicine formally became a medical specialty. Since the early 1980s, the government has established research units and now every institute for family medicine also has a research unit attached. Academic family medicine has gradually grown to include 15 professors and a large number of PhD students, post-doctoral researchers and senior researchers by 2015.

CURRENT ACTIVITY

Danish research in family medicine has developed from basic descriptive research into using highly advanced study designs including intervention studies acknowledging the often-complex trajectories in general practice. Thus, many research projects now include qualitative and quantitative research methods. Further, the research also focuses on the interplay between clinical work, health services research and implementation.

Out-of-hours primary care and acute care

Denmark has a long tradition of research on how first-line primary care best provides out-of-hours care and serves the public regarding acute care. This exploration includes clinical research, epidemiology and interventions with different provider organisations.

Health checks and screening for lifestyle diseases

Family medicine plays an important role in prevention of lifestyle diseases. The questions are how prevention is best organised to render results and how to avoid potential adverse effects. Danish research is based on large national and international projects including intervention studies, especially in diabetes care. Important aspects are how to avoid unintended harmful consequences of care; not stigmatising healthy citizens by introducing fearful perceptions of their own health (overdiagnosis); and how to avoid 'too much medicine', both in terms of diagnostics and treatment.

Diagnosis in primary care

Family medicine is the place where citizens present with symptoms for the first time. The GP must know exactly how these symptoms should be interpreted, investigated and how often they might be a sign of serious disease. A research focus on patients' care pathway, from their first symptom until treatment, has been initiated. It involves aspects of clinical, organisational and behavioural research. Thus, a part of it involves how the public experiences symptoms, how often and why these symptoms lead to healthcare seeking and how symptoms affect clinical decision-making. Issues of increasing use of technology and risk assessment are included in the understanding of patients, their practices and their interactions with the frontline of our healthcare systems.

Mental disease and multi-morbidity

One emerging part of family medicine research in Denmark concerns mental illness in general practice and the fact that the care and prognosis is poor, in particular due to physical multi-morbidity. This also includes children's mental health. The research includes advanced epidemiological studies on the role of general practice, prognosis and intervention studies integrating all parts of the healthcare system.

GAINS AND CHALLENGES
Cancer pathways in primary care

Research showed the long waiting time from first symptom until treatment and resulted in national health system implementation of 'urgent referral for cancer suspicion'.[15] It has been further developed and now forms a generic frame for a so-called three-legged strategy for diagnosis of all serious disease in general practice. The challenge is that there is an urgent need for better knowledge on which investigations should be rationally applied to ensure optimal use of resources and, particularly, finding the right balance with relation to identifying possible pathologies with no immediate impact on the patients' health.

Integrated psychiatric care

Based on the need for better diagnostic pathways, earlier treatment and long-term follow-up, an integration of psychiatric care has started. Use of fast track diagnostic assessment and stepped care is now being implemented.

Data collection, security and availability

An important part of the research development has been the focus on infrastructure and data availability. The Danish health system registers a large amount of data that can be linked to the individual through a personal identifier. During the last decade, general practice developed a comprehensive and innovative data collection system based on electronic data capture. These data were used for quality assurance and research. The technology developed was, in an international context, ground breaking. The challenge is to ensure optimal data protection and safety and that data are used only for the right purpose.

FUTURE DIRECTIONS
Avoiding inequity in health through primary care

Combatting the 'inverse care law', in which healthy, resourceful citizens get too much care, thereby hindering and limiting the provision of care for those in need. What is the role of general practice, and how will increased use of resources for multi-morbidity and new treatments affect the work in general practice?

Priority setting in primary care

The pressure from the public and from technological development will, in a gatekeeper-based system, lead to an even higher responsibility placed on general practice.[15] The priorities of activities in general practice will have a huge impact on the healthcare system as a whole, and general practice will need tools to ensure that priority setting is based on evidence.

Providing high medical quality in an affordable healthcare system

The importance of general practice to ensure an affordable healthcare system is evident. The questions are: how do we invest in primary care; what is the right skills mix; and how do we best integrate this mix with the rest of the healthcare system, maintaining the right balance between what is managed in primary care and what needs referral? Issues of access, quality, safety and cost-effectiveness will all need to be based on primary care research.

CHAPTER 29

Primary care research in Spain

. . . .

Sergio Minué

HISTORY

The specialty of family and community medicine was only established in Spain in 1979, and primary care research output has generally been very low, at only 0.6% of the total biomedical research production between 1985 and 2008.[16]

Major advances since 1979 include the creation of a specific medical specialty for primary care, known as 'family and community medicine', as well as the establishment of Family Medicine Teaching Units (FMTUs). The role of the FMTU is to train future family physicians in research methods appropriate to the specific context of primary healthcare and to promote research projects by primary care professionals. Currently, most of the research (66%) is performed within health centres.[17]

In addition, the Spanish Society of Family and Community Medicine (semFYC) initiated a scientific journal entitled *Atención Primaria*, which subsequently published almost 40% of primary care research in the period 2000–2009, although, currently, this has fallen to only 22.5%.[17]

Further advances centre on the establishment of research networks:[18]

- Research units networks in some primary healthcare districts, such as Red de Unidades de Investigación in the 1990s.
- The Research Network on Preventive Activities and Health Promotion (REDIAPP), since 2003.
- The Biomedical Research Network (CIBER).
- The experience from Seminars of Innovation on Primary Care (SIAP) since 2005, led by the CESCA group, which promotes informal collaboration networking in the field of implementation research. The name arises from the first publicly funded project in 1984, 'Correlacion entre las Entradas y las Salidas en la Consulta Ambulatoria' (Correlation between Inputs and Outputs in Ambulatory Consultation).

CURRENT ACTIVITY

Current primary care research activity focuses on the following four areas:

1. Prevalent clinical problems, with special attention to chronic diseases (cardiovascular diseases, mental health, endocrine and infectious diseases) and multi-morbidity.
2. Prevention, health promotion and lifestyle.
3. Health services, especially regarding the effectiveness and efficiency of new organisational models, financing systems, professional payment systems and primary care assessment.
4. Clinical decision-making in primary care.

GAINS AND CHALLENGES

Currently, Spain ranks second, after the UK, in the absolute number and percentage of scientific publications on primary care among European countries and seventh in terms of the number of papers per million inhabitants. The increase in scientific production has been slow, but steady, from 170 in 2008 to 291 in 2012.[16] There was also an increase in the number of publications in journals with an impact factor that is measurable by Journal Citation Report (JCR)®. Currently, these publications have a mean impact factor of 1.7 and a median of 1.3.[19] Research networks have also been consolidated, in some cases with colleagues and institutions from other countries.

However, primary care research has not yet reached the critical volume, quality, relevance or desirable impact, and key factors responsible for this include the absence of university departments of primary care and therefore engagement with primary care in the academic context.[18] In addition, low levels of funding for primary care research projects is a challenge. Funding from the National Research Agency has progressively declined, from 122 primary care projects in 2005 to only 20 in 2013, which represents just 3% of all projects funded.

FUTURE DIRECTIONS

1. New research networks focus on population health, health services research and clinical practice (REDIAPP, CIBER, SIAP). The current project from semFYC to get a Spanish map of primary care researchers may be a useful contribution. These initiatives should be complemented by specific supportive research structures and the availability of time to research.
2. A specific field of knowledge that is regarded as the focus of primary care research should be outlined through research and implementation projects. Some examples of this could be projects that focus on clinical decision-making under uncertainty, time and continuity as diagnostic strategies in primary care, the process of illness, the holistic approach to patients and not diseases, the social and community determinants of disease, the effectiveness of non-pharmacological interventions or the analysis of health-seeking behaviour that encourages overdiagnosis and

overtreatment, and protecting the population from unnecessary interventions through quaternary prevention.[20]

3. The establishment of partnerships with professionals, universities and research units from other countries, taking advantage of the privileged position of Spain, which straddles both Europe and America, and allows the establishment of joint projects with researchers on both sides of the Atlantic Ocean.

CHAPTER 30

Primary care research in Turkey

. . . .

Mehmet Akman

HISTORY

Family medicine is a relatively young academic discipline in Turkey. Primary care services were exclusively provided by medical graduates with no vocational training up until 1985, when the first training positions in family medicine became available at tertiary teaching hospitals. Establishment of family medicine departments at universities started in 1993, and the first associate professor who completed family medicine vocational training was appointed in 1996.[21] Since then, the number of academics in the field has increased rapidly, with 32 professors and 72 associate professors by December 2014. The Higher Education Council of Turkey has mandated that academic promotion requires a minimum of three published articles, which should be in journals indexed by the Science Citation Index Expanded. Since this rule has come into effect, there has been a clear increase in the number of scientific publications originating from Turkey, although often in relatively low impact factor journals.

CURRENT ACTIVITY

Currently, there are 63 departments of family medicine all over the country that play an active role in both undergraduate and postgraduate medical teaching.[22] These numbers indicate a significant research capacity for primary care research. Accordingly, the number of scientific national journals in the field of family medicine has increased gradually in recent years. Besides the leading *Turkish Journal of Family Practice*, which is owned by the Turkish Family Medicine Association (TAHUD) and was established in 1997, there are 10 other primary care journals publishing original research papers, systematic reviews or translated research articles.

Several regional and national family medicine meetings, which act as platforms for the presentation of primary care research, take place on a regular basis. Among these, the top three are The National Congress organised by TAHUD, the Autumn School organised by the Turkish Family Medicine Foundation and the biannual Primary Care Research Days organised by the Family Medicine Academicians Association. In 2014, there were 773 research presentations split between these events.

Turkish family medicine academics are widely represented in international networks, associations and other organisations. The European General Practice Research Network (EGPRN), working under the umbrella of the World Organization of Family Doctors (WONCA) Europe, is the most crucial one for primary care researchers in Europe. This network has more than 20 active and regular Turkish members, and, as of December 2014, three of the EGPRN biannual conferences have taken place in Turkey.

GAINS AND CHALLENGES

Over the last decade, the Health Transformation Programme (HTP) was gradually introduced in Turkey to reform the national public health system. One of the important components of this programme was the introduction of a family medicine scheme. Despite all the structural and procedural reforms associated with the HTP, the Primary Health Care Activity Monitor for Europe rated the structure of primary care as 'medium', and the primary care service delivery process as 'weak' in Turkey compared with other countries in Europe.[23] The major issues for stronger primary care in Turkey were a lack of comprehensive and coordinated care, insufficient human resources for health and poor multidisciplinary teamwork.[24]

Medical graduates with no vocational training still provide more than 90% of primary care services and have limited research capacity. Additional challenges to primary care research include a lack of funding, bureaucratic obstacles to accessing primary care data and few academic primary care centres. The latter restricts the patient care provided by family medicine academicians only to teaching hospitals.

FUTURE DIRECTIONS

The development of academic family medicine departments within the last 20 years is at a level comparable with many countries in Europe. The most important priority of the family medicine departments in the next 10 years is to establish academic teaching practices and strengthen the relations with family physicians on the ground.[22] New legislation introduced in 2014 allows academic units to establish primary care centres at which they can train family physicians outside of teaching hospitals. The establishment of academic primary care centres within communities will enhance the capacity to build research networks and coordinate primary care research.

International collaboration is another important way to increase the quality and quantity of primary care research. The Quality and Costs of Primary Care in Europe (QUALICOPC) study, which aims to evaluate the performance of primary care systems in Europe in terms of quality, equity and costs, is a good example of such collaboration.[25] Results of this study will give us a better insight into Turkish primary care in the context of the HTP and guide us in terms of which areas need improvement.

The overall challenge is to conduct good-quality primary care research that would have an impact on both practice and policy levels with a view to developing a stronger Turkish primary care system. The EGPRN research agenda[26] is a good framework that can be used to determine priorities based on the country's needs.

Eastern Mediterranean Region

CHAPTER 31

Primary care research in Israel

. . . .

Khaled Karkabi

HISTORY

Israel initiated postgraduate residency training for family medicine (FM) in 1969 and therefore became one of the first seven countries accepted for membership in the World Organization of Family Doctors (WONCA).[27] Research in primary care (PC) in Israel developed alongside the growth of FM as an academic discipline. The following are milestones in the development of research in PC in Israel:

1. Jack Medalie, the founder of the Department of Family Medicine at Tel Aviv University, Israel, and later at Case Western Reserve University in Cleveland, Ohio, USA, was a world pioneer in cardiovascular epidemiology. Together with colleagues and funding from the National Institutes of Health, he conducted the Israel Ischemic Heart Disease Study in 1963 to analyse factors having a positive or negative correlation with ischemic heart disease. The study population of 10 000 male civil servants living in Israel, aged 40–75, was followed for 23 years. The variables under scrutiny focused on six areas: genetic, socio-demographic, clinical, biochemical, behavioural and psychosocial. The study results were published in more than 100 papers in leading medical journals.[28]
2. RAMBAM, the Family Medicine Research Network in Israel, was founded in 1991 to encourage research in PC and the advancement of family physicians' academic achievements.[29] This resulted in improving the organisation and nature of the

research in PC and led to the publication of several major studies. Among others, studies on sexual abuse and low back pain were conducted. One of the founders of the research network is Jeffrey Borkan, later the chair of the Department of Family Medicine at Brown University in Providence, Rhode Island, USA.[30]

3. The Sial Research Centre at Ben-Gurion University, founded in 2000, has contributed to research in PC in Israel, in general, and to the national palliative care training programme and family practice and health policy in PC, in particular.

4. The Israel National Institute for Health Policy Research (NIHP) is another independent organisation, which strives to promote and fund research pertaining to the economics, quality of services and decision-making processes in the health system in Israel. To date, the NIHP has funded dozens of studies on health policy, organisation of healthcare services, health economics and the quality of national healthcare services.

CURRENT ACTIVITY

PC research conducted by the departments of FM in the country, and the topics it encompasses, is diverse. Research funding in PC comes from varied sources. The Israel Association of Family Physicians, home to more than 2000 members, encourages and supports research by allocating annual grants to the finest research proposals. The NIHP, as mentioned earlier, and the Clalit health maintenance organisations (HMOs) also allocate a substantial annual budget for research in the community.

The most salient current PC research activities include:

1. Health services in the community: by law, Israel provides health insurance for all. Since the late 1990s, PC records have been completely converted to electronic medical records, creating excellent, up-to-date data on population health, utilisation of health services and healthcare givers, thus making it one of the best in the world. Research in health services covers a wide range of topics: quality in PC, adherence to treatment,[31] chronic disease management,[32,33] mental illness[34] and the organisation of PC services.

2. Palliative care and pain management: for nearly two decades, the Department of Family Medicine at Ben-Gurion University has been developing palliative care in the Negev.[35] The goal for the next few years is to extend the services to areas not currently receiving them and to further improve the existing services. Research is conducted on chronic pain in the community, including the prevalence of patients suffering from chronic pain, estimation and evaluation of the different treatments and the organisation of pain care in the community.[36]

3. Studies of attitudes and practices of both caregivers and patients encompassing a wide range of conditions.

GAINS AND CHALLENGES

Healthcare in the community is delivered by four HMOs, with Clalit Health Services, the largest one, providing coverage for more than half of the population. This well-organised healthcare system, which introduced nationwide comprehensive electronic medical records 20 years ago, is an excellent potential resource for research in PC, including:

1. Research based on PC electronic data: during the last few years there has been an abundance of research on the epidemiology of illness in the community, chronic disease management, interaction between medication and various diseases and the use of technology in healthcare.
2. Research on health services, caregivers and patients in PC: in an era when the number of physicians is insufficient, and strains on healthcare budgets are increasing, it is vital to explore how PC can tackle these challenges and find the best ways in which to deliver healthcare.

FUTURE DIRECTIONS

Future research should address problems encountered in PC and improve healthcare. I would like to emphasise the following topics:

1. Health services, including the provision of team work in PC: the strains and overload on primary care physicians (PCPs) have reached a point which warrants implementing new methods of work in PC. Probably the biggest challenge will be to restore teamwork in PC clinics, which was terminated about 20 years ago due to budget constraints. In a rapidly changing world, involving massive technological developments, the public's needs from, and expectations of, PCPs should be reassessed and formalised. The same applies to PCPs' views and perceptions of their role in the community.
2. Research on multi-morbidity: how the Israeli healthcare system should deal with the growing demands of the elderly population with multiple morbidity.
3. Adherence to treatment: this has become a popular research topic worldwide; the cultural and economic diversity of Israeli society poses additional challenges in studies aimed at improving patients' adherence to treatment.
4. Palliative and pain care in the community: due to the ageing of the population, the need for more palliative and pain care is evident. Research should focus on delving more deeply into the prevalence of the problems and challenges, as well as various holistic treatment modalities and cost-efficient methods of care.

CHAPTER 32

Primary care research in the Kingdom of Bahrain

....

Faisal Abdullatif Alnasir

HISTORY

Primary healthcare (PHC) services have been available in the Kingdom of Bahrain for more than 40 years.[37] These services were provided by non-specialised general practitioners within primary healthcare centres across the country. In 1981, a decision was taken by the minister of health to start a structured training programme for doctors called the Family Practice Residency Program (FPRP). The programme aimed at graduating qualified family physicians (FPs) who would shoulder the responsibility of providing quality PHC services to the population.[38]

The first medical school in the Kingdom, the College of Medicine and Medical Sciences (CMMS) of the Arabian Gulf University, was established in 1983, and, a few years later, two further medical colleges were founded. Since the beginning, the CMMS adopted problem-based learning methods within a community-oriented curriculum that emphasised PHC, family medicine and research. The CMMS also played a major role in promoting research among its medical students and faculty.[39-41] One of the most important activities within the CMMS Department of Family and Community Medicine is community-oriented research. This programme extends over 1 year and is aimed at teaching research methodology to medical students who are required to do research at an undergraduate level. Many doctors from the Ministry of Health (MOH) were appointed as part-time faculty in the CMMS to provide clinical training and teaching. To be accepted in the academic hierarchy and promoted, they are also required to engage with research and publish their work.

On the other hand, although the FPRP residents were initially oriented to the subject of research, it only became mandatory for each resident (in groups) to think about a topic and implement a research study during their training period in 1990.

With these two developments, the FPRP and the CMMS, more and more attention was given to the subject of primary care research. This was in addition to the emergence of two medical journals, the *Bahrain Medical Bulletin* (in 1979) and the *Journal of the Bahrain Medical Society* (more than 20 years ago), which played a significant role in increasing research awareness and skills of medical professionals.

The MOH has also created regulations to enhance research activities among its doctors and allow doctors to be promoted from one rank to another (e.g. to consultant and senior consultant level). Research publications have also become a requirement.

CURRENT ACTIVITY

Currently, within the MOH, a research committee, with a sub-committee for PHC, has been established. The main objectives of these committees are to increase the awareness of the medical staff about the importance of research, encourage them to do research, provide help and assistance to those interested, supervise the research quality and ensure that related ethical issues and patients' safety are taken care of.

The FPRP curriculum has also been enriched with a structured teaching module on research at the beginning of the course (in year 1) for which they are taught research fundamentals, epidemiology, evidence-based medicine and given information about the Cochrane Library.[42] Residents are then required to choose a research question, submit a protocol, do a pilot study and implement their research. In the final year of their training period, they are required to write up their results, submit their final product and make the work ready for publication.[43]

GAINS AND CHALLENGES

Once the residents graduate from the FPRP, they are appointed as FPs in the PHC centres that are distributed around the country. FPs who are engaged in research and have published papers are promoted to FP specialists and receive priority for attending conferences. Such action has helped in increasing the number of published research articles from Bahrain.

Increased awareness of research and its implementation has contributed to the quality of health services and the health of the population. This has been reflected in:

- The upgrading of PHC services.
- Improvement of the FPs' clinical and prescription-writing skills.[44]
- More use of evidence-based medicine in FPs' practice.
- More FPs conducting regular audits for quality assurance.
- The increased health awareness of the public.
- A reduction in the prevalence of communicable and non-communicable as well as hereditary blood diseases.
- Improvement of the training and teaching methods in the FPRP.

There are many challenges faced that may hinder the full-scale implementation of research policies within PHC; among the most important are:

- Lack of funds assigned to support research.
- No dedicated time for FPs to do research in their busy schedule.
- The marginalisation of research activities and loss of interest from the small number of FPs who must deliver the services.
- A lack of commitment from some policymakers and managers to include research in the job description of FPs.

FUTURE DIRECTIONS

In the long term, research has to be strengthened in the Kingdom to impact the many health problems such as hereditary blood diseases, non-communicable diseases and obesity. There are many opportunities that could help in promoting research in the country. Among the most important are:

- A strong Family and Community Medicine Council, as part of the Arab Board for Health specialities, which is overlooking the teaching, training and qualification of FPs in the Arab world.
- All medical schools in the country and in the region have an established department of family medicine.
- Many primary care and family medicine conferences are organised in the region.
- Many large organisations, such as the World Organization of Family Doctors and the World Health Organization Regional Office for the Eastern Mediterranean, are supportive of primary care research.
- The practising FPs are required to be engaged in continuing professional development with a minimum number of credit hours per year that includes research.
- Various non-government and private agencies are providing grants for research.[45]
- The *Bahrain Medical Bulletin* awards annual prizes for the best research done in the country.[46]

South Asia Region

CHAPTER 33

Primary care research in India

....

Raman Kumar

HISTORY

Within academic circles and in practice, the term 'primary care' is considered synonymous with 'public health' in India. Disease-focused vertical programmes have remained the mainstay of primary care delivery in this, the second most populous country in the world. Medical doctors are an important and desirable component of primary care teams in the form of (1) medical officers in the public sector and (2) general practitioners in the private sector. However, their role has remained limited to that of a 'basic' doctor without any academic or research opportunities.

Since the 1980s, departments of preventive and social medicine (PSM; also called community medicine [CM]) were introduced to medical colleges in India under the Re-Orientation of Medical Education (ROME) programme, to facilitate implementation of public health measures and vertical programmes. Public health and primary care research has been traditionally delegated to these departments.

CURRENT ACTIVITY

In spite of the best of intentions, these departments have not evolved to their fullest potential, and their role has been limited to medical public health, as they are dominated by the medical profession. These academic departments of PSM/CM have not managed to create a significant research output and remain somewhat dysfunctional in this regard. There is a recent trend to re-designate PSM/CM departments as schools of public health to allow the development of public health in its broader meaning. Recognition of a separate and distinct discipline of primary care, family medicine or general practice is a relatively recent phenomenon. In the absence of any distinct academic departments for primary care or family medicine, primary care research is underdeveloped in India.

GAINS AND CHALLENGES

The Department of Health Research (DHR), under the Ministry of Health and Family Welfare, is the umbrella government organisation that coordinates and facilitates all research activities in the health sector. The Indian Council for Medical Research is the principal funding agency for medical research, functioning under the DHR. The other funding agencies are the Department of Science and Technology, the Central Council for Scientific and Industrial Research and the Department of Biotechnology. However, in the absence of formal academic family medicine and primary care departments, funding utilisation towards primary care research is limited. There are also some limited funding opportunities from the private sector for public health and primary care research.

Within the public health domain, there has been a spurt of research activities in the last decade. The main areas of public health research are population-based surveys and health programme evaluations. Analysis of research papers in the public health domain reveals that many of the high-morbidity disease conditions are underrepresented. The Public Health Foundation of India (PHFI), launched in 2006, is spearheading public health education and research in India. During the past decade, the PHFI has undertaken several research initiatives and consultancy projects, which underline the healthcare reforms and gradual movement towards universal health coverage.

There are several non-governmental organisations as well that undertake public health education and research in India. According to an analysis of public health research papers in India, the majority were epidemiological and few focused on health policy and systems.[47] Several major causes of the disease burden in India continue to be underrepresented in the quality-adjusted public health research output.

Due to lack of governance, infrastructure and funding in primary care, the following are important areas of concern:

1. The absence of robust mechanisms for ethical clearance and administrative support in primary care research.
2. The lack of reliable morbidity data for populations – most of the data available in the public domain are indirect estimates.
3. Clinical guidelines are either based on tertiary care research or adopted international guidelines with little input from primary care.
4. There are few case reports from community settings, which could be epidemiologically relevant.
5. The lack of quality and standards in primary care due to the absence of clinical audits and quality improvement studies.
6. The impact assessment of public health intervention (or programmes) may be flawed.

7. Public health budgeting is skewed towards donor interests and vertical programmes.

FUTURE DIRECTIONS

Promotion of family medicine as a distinct academic discipline has been supported by several policy documents by the Government of India, including the *National Health Policy 2002*.[48] Family medicine has been a recognised postgraduate qualification since 1983 by the National Board of Examination (NBE); however, full-time residency training in family medicine only began in the last decade. Currently, there are 65 recognised training centres in India, which are accredited by the NBE (running postgraduate programmes only) with a capacity for 200 residents per annum. The residents train for the Diploma of the National Board in Family Medicine. At present, these residencies are organised under the specialist faculty and mostly in hospital settings. Within the mainstream medical education system, under the Medical Council of India, the first postgraduate MD in family medicine course was established at Calicut Medical College, Kerala, in 2012. The Christian Medical College, Vellore, has also established a fully functional independent academic department of family medicine and is currently in the process of starting an MD family medicine programme. As a compulsory requirement towards the award of this postgraduate qualification, residents have to undertake a research project and submit a thesis towards the end of their residency training.

In 2012, the *Journal of Family Medicine and Primary Care*, the first dedicated peer-reviewed primary care journal, was established.

In the wake of the Government of India's ambition to implement universal health coverage, it is of utmost importance that primary care research be encouraged and supported. However, this requires simultaneous efforts to strengthen the academic departments of family medicine at all medical colleges in India.

CHAPTER 34

Primary care research in Pakistan

....

Tabinda Ashfaq

HISTORY

Medical research had its formal inception in 1962 when the Pakistan Medical Research Council (PMRC) was created as an autonomous organisation under the Federal Ministry of Health. The major mandate of the PMRC was to promote, organise and coordinate medical research in Pakistan. The College of Family Medicine, a college for the growth and development of family physicians, was established in 1974 and became a World Organization of Family Doctors (WONCA) member the same year. However, not much work was done in research until 2010, when the WONCA Working Party on Research started functioning on an active basis for the professional growth and enhancement of research activities among general practitioners.

CURRENT ACTIVITY

Several organisations are working for family physicians'/general practitioners' professional development and capacity building in the area of medicine and research in Pakistan. These include the College of Family Medicine, the WONCA Working Party on Research, the Pakistan Academy of Family Physicians and the South Asian Primary Care Research Network. All of these organisations are working to improve clinical knowledge, promote primary care research in the region and build capacity to achieve these objectives and, ultimately, to improve the healthcare system of Pakistan. They have been actively involved in organising lectures, workshops and conferences and promoting a research culture in primary care. They have also been involved in mentoring family physicians to publish research in different scientific journals, although the number of published works is currently very low.[49] In 2014, a research workshop was organised by the South Asian Primary Care Research Network and the WONCA Working Party on Research for general practitioners. This was well received, and a mentorship programme has subsequently been started in which senior family physicians are paired with junior physicians to facilitate research activities. A number of collaborative research projects have been initiated to develop networking and improve health status in the region.

The Spice Route Movement is a WONCA South Asia Region working group for new and future doctors who have an interest in family/general practice.[50] It facilitates young doctors to grow professionally and participate in family medicine conferences. The main aim is the promotion of excellence in the field of family medicine / general practice in order to respond to growing health challenges. The Higher Education Commission has also promoted research activities through scholarships and grants; although the number of people supported is limited due to a scarcity of resources.

GAINS AND CHALLENGES

Although research on the common conditions seen in Pakistan primary care would strengthen the health system and be of social value, such research is currently rudimentary. With the help of the mentioned organisations and groups, there is a growing culture of research in primary care. As a result, family physicians understand the need for and importance of research in primary care, particularly that targeting chronic illnesses; however, there is still a long way to go. Vocational training does not focus on research capacity and therefore family physicians have little expertise or motivation to engage with research. Furthermore, medical colleges and universities do not have research-friendly environments, and medical students are not encouraged to participate in research activities.[51] Other barriers and obstacles to overcome include limited knowledge, the busy schedule of general practitioners, the limited availability of funds, limited resources, language barriers and poor guidance.[52]

FUTURE DIRECTIONS

Pakistan faces a double burden of infectious and non-communicable diseases, with the major burden being from conditions such as diabetes, hypertension and dyslipidaemia. More research is required to understand and respond to these challenges in community settings and primary care. Research in primary care is essential to develop and implement clinical guidelines that will improve clinical practice. Research should be designed to develop cost-effective interventions that impact on local health indicators and can be taken to scale nationally. The poor health indicators in Pakistan suggest a more urgent commitment is needed to the contribution that primary care research can make to strengthen the health system.

Asia Pacific Region

CHAPTER 35

Primary care research in China

....

William Wong

HISTORY

Since gaining power in 1949, a top priority for the new communist China has been controlling rampant epidemics of fatal infectious diseases. The government wisely adopted a primary care system approach that integrated public health. Remarkable achievements were made to the national health status and acclaimed by the World Health Organization (WHO) as 'a unique model for developing countries'.[53] The Rural Community Medical Service, barefoot doctors, and three levels of healthcare networks are just a few programmes from the 1960s and 1970s. However, market-oriented reforms in 1978 left people suffering poor access to healthcare and poor healthcare services, as primary care was replaced by market-led specialty care, until the reintroduction of health reforms in 1998.[54]

At the beginning of the economic reform, the healthcare authorities and researchers overlooked the key role of government and the unique nature of the healthcare sector. It was believed that, like other economy sectors, it would thrive in a market-oriented environment on its own accord. This has been proved fundamentally mistaken. It is now recognised that the central government plays a crucial role, from healthcare policymaking to financial support to healthcare workforce training. Central government policies dictate the landscape of healthcare. Its investment is key to the success of any sustainable healthcare system.

CURRENT ACTIVITY

The most important development is revived interest in primary healthcare and improved understanding of the concept of 'family medicine / general practice' (FM). The essence of this (such as the '5 Cs' and '10 principles') has been recognised by scholars and officials,[55] and many experimental community health centres and rural township hospitals which also provided family medicine services were set up across China. The importance of training a large workforce of family doctors was implemented in the late 1990s – for instance, the 5yrs + 3yrs GP structured vocational training programme in urban areas, and the 3yrs + 2yrs rural GP structured vocational training programme in rural areas. Nonetheless, little primary care medical education is evidence based. Medical education research is not high priority in Chinese medical research.

The *Chinese Journal of General Practice* conducted an analysis of its publications in 2014 which revealed that the majority focused on health policies, healthcare and medical education – for example, integration of primary care into the healthcare system. Researchers of certain medical specialities focused on improving care for specific patients, with less attention paid to providing care at the personal/consultation level.

GAINS AND CHALLENGES

The most exciting and unique feature of China's primary care research is the prominence of specialists from other disciplines actively supporting research on and development of primary care. Yet for a discipline to be truly independent, research must address discipline-specific questions. FM research should engage with the complexity of signs, symptoms and psychosocial issues that arise from the primary care context. Family doctors need research to guide them in making effective evidence-based clinical decisions in this context, within the constraints of the healthcare system. These clinical and related research questions are not necessarily appreciated or addressed by other hospital-based specialists.

Two main challenges for developing primary care research in the current healthcare system are:

1. Establishing sustainable systems to attract trained doctors into primary care in township hospitals and community centres. This should involve rewarding work with salaries comparable to those obtainable in cities. Following this, incentives should be provided to these physicians to take on research projects. An encouraging development is the new 2014 'special job posts' experimental programme for general practitioners, and the current requirement to complete a research project for promotion to a senior position.
2. Building research capacity and resources. Gradually, more medical universities, including Fudan University and Peking University, are establishing general practice departments and actively seeking government support and investments to develop primary care. The large influence of these institutions to fuel teaching and research

makes this a significant development in primary care. However, building capacity and resources are significant issues, as primary care research is still not a key area of development.

FUTURE DIRECTIONS

General practitioner-centred residency training programmes that include research training and evidence utilisation must be established for current and future generations of family doctors. This is key to providing high-quality care for all populations under the notion of universal care, especially in the fast-paced medical arena.

One potential area of primary care research would be providing high-quality and accessible universal care across urban and rural regions. Active research and experiments in primary care to attract family doctors to work in the countryside are essential. Incentives, such as overseas registration, scholarships or additional support, have been used in other countries.

Another would be to address allocation of healthcare resources from tertiary to primary care, and meeting the core roles of primary healthcare by attracting, advancing and rewarding clinicians for high quality practice should be explored. A fair and rewarding job and promotions comparable to those for specialty physicians are fundamental. Evidence is needed to convince the central government of cost-effectiveness and potential health improvements, helping to generate necessary funds for development and supporting the ultimate goal to achieve universal care.

Currently, most of China's healthcare centres and township hospitals have poor performance and poor-quality research, lacking efficient management systems and capacity. Earmarked funding, more directives on research and collaborations with established universities are needed. The sheer number of family doctors in China who could potentially be involved in primary care research would make a significant force in the field.

CHAPTER 36

Primary care research in Malaysia

....

Sherina Mohd Sidik

HISTORY

The most important developments in primary care research in Malaysia since 1960 have been in the (1) identification of priority research areas, (2) development of the Family Medicine Specialist Training Programme and (3) increase in number of publications.

Malaysia had a total of 65 hospitals when it gained independence in 1957, and post-independence, the government focused on improving the socioeconomic development of its population. From 1957 to 1977, the national healthcare system focused on developing and upgrading its primary healthcare services.[56] The focus changed from communicable diseases (infectious diseases) to non-communicable diseases (NCDs), as cardiovascular diseases, cancer and mental health disorders became more prevalent in Malaysia from the 1990s.[57]

The first documented evidence of primary care research in Malaysia was a publication on haemoptysis in 1966.[58] In *Bibliography of Primary Care Research in Malaysia*, 1222 papers were identified from 1966 to 2003. Most papers were mainly on infectious diseases from the 1960s to 1990s. However, from mid-1990, papers on endocrine/metabolic/nutrition, general symptoms, occupational health, psychological, respiratory and pregnancy-related disorders were also found.[58]

Since 1993, Malaysia has achieved comprehensive healthcare services at the primary care level. The Family Medicine Specialist Training Program at Malaysian government universities was fully supported by the Ministry of Health (MOH) to ensure the continuation of this achievement. The specialty of family medicine was established with a 4-year master's course in 1993.[56] Family medicine specialists (FMSs) started working in health clinics in 1997 to improve quality of primary care. Currently, there are 218 FMSs, heading 918 primary care clinics in 13 states and two federal territories in Malaysia.[59]

Many FMSs who joined the Malaysian government universities as lecturers have been pursuing their PhD studies nationally and internationally, which has contributed to the advancement of primary care research. In 2009, the Public Service Department approved doctors working in the MOH for master's and doctoral degrees. This increased the training of FMSs in the MOH in research as well.[59]

The number of publications in primary care research has increased significantly in Malaysia from 1960 till today. The number of publications increased from 92 (1966–1975) to 220 (1976–1985) to 375 (1986–1995) and to 507 (1996–2003).[58] A search conducted of the Scopus database on November 2014 showed that there were 85 publications on primary care research in Malaysia from 1969 to 2014, and 54 (60.35%) of these were published from the year 2000 onwards.

CURRENT ACTIVITY

The most salient current primary care research activity in Malaysia, based on the top 20 publications in the past three years (2012–2014), is:

1. Randomised controlled trials and qualitative studies on interventions for non-communicable diseases.
2. On health promotion services in primary care.
3. On current management of diseases in primary care.

The study designs in primary care research in Malaysia have improved from case series to cross-sectional studies, progressing to case-control studies, cohort studies and clinical trials. Based on the *Bibliography of Primary Care Research in Malaysia*, most papers from 1966 to 2003 were either case series (11.9%) or cross-sectional (62.0%) studies. There were very few analytical observational studies; case-control studies (3.4%), clinical trials (4.1%), cohort studies (1.3%) and qualitative studies (0.7%).[58]

However, from 2003 onwards, there has been an upgrade of research designs in Malaysia in line with the establishment of the Clinical Research Centre (CRC) in 2000. The CRC functions as the clinical research arm of the MOH and assists in establishing research protocol, research project planning, project management and publication. It specifically focuses on clinical trials in line with Malaysia's Third Industrial Master Plan 2006–2020.[60]

GAINS AND CHALLENGES

The greatest primary care research capability in Malaysia now lies with the FMSs in universities and MOH.

The important thing being achieved is the development of research in new areas of primary care. FMSs are being trained overseas and locally in various areas such as NCDs, substance abuse, community psychiatry, community paediatrics and community geriatrics. FMSs are now improving health services in primary care in these areas.

The big challenges are in:

1. Establishing good collaboration between universities and the MOH in terms of

research development. The university FMSs have knowledge and expertise in conducting research in various areas of primary care. However, they need to utilise patients and healthcare services in government primary care clinics and outpatient departments in government hospitals, which are under the administration of the MOH.

2. Obtaining sufficient funds to conduct larger and more in-depth studies. Grants are now being awarded for research that focuses on the outcome of an intervention in priority areas highlighted by the MOH.

FUTURE DIRECTIONS

The three most promising and important opportunities for further primary care research in Malaysia are:

1. *Collaboration with the Institute of Public Health (IPH) Malaysia and CRC*
   Malaysia's current strategy is for research development and internationalisation through networking with various international research centres and institutes. Other than the CRC, the IPH is also conducting research projects with other agencies including the World Health Organization and the Centers for Disease Control and Prevention, Atlanta, Georgia, USA.[60] By collaborating with the IPH and CRC, primary care research in Malaysia is developing towards research that will be internationally recognised.

2. *Contribution to the Clinical Practice Guidelines (CPGs) by the Health Technology Assessment, MOH*
   CPGs in Malaysia provide accurate management strategies for various diseases in the Malaysian community. These management guidelines are based on evidence obtained from national and international research and publications.[61] Contribution to CPGs will enable FMSs to provide evidence-based medicine in the management of diseases in primary care.

3. *The development of the Malaysian Primary Care Research Group (MPCRG)*
   The MPCRG[62] was developed in 2004 under the Academy of Family Physicians Malaysia (AFPM).[63] The AFPM's Member of AFPM / Fellow of The Royal Australian College of General Practitioners Vocational Training Programme includes research in its training curriculum and provides an opportunity for research among general practitioners, the MOH and universities. In line with this training programme, the MPCRG has conducted 13 workshops and also initiated the inaugural Asia Pacific Primary Care Research Conference in 2009.[62]

CHAPTER 37

Primary care research in Australia

· ·

Ellen McIntyre

HISTORY

General practice research in Australia began formally with the establishment in the mid-1970s of academic departments of community medicine that subsequently morphed into departments of general practice.[64] Primary care research was further supported in the mid-1980s with the founding of the professional organisation the Australian Association of Academic General Practice, now named the Australasian Association of Academic Primary Care to better reflect the organisation's membership (30% are non–general practitioners [GPs]) and the inclusion of New Zealand PHC (PHC) researchers. In the early 2000s, The Royal Australian College of General Practitioners (RACGP) also enhanced its focus on research through the Standing Committee on Research and the RACGP Research Foundation.

Federal government funding specific to research in general practice was provided via the General Practice Evaluation Program, operating in the 1990s. This programme funded 248 projects, 13% of which were interventions studies.[65]

Since 2000, the federal government has invested over $135 million in PHC research funding via the Primary Health Care Research, Evaluation and Development (PHCRED) Strategy to 'build the primary health care research capacity and evidence base, in order to improve health outcomes through better primary health care systems, services and practices'.[66] While this includes primary care research, it also encompasses broader PHC research.

Between 2000 and 2011, university departments of general practice and rural health (established in the 1990s) received PHCRED funding to build research capacity and conduct relevant high-quality research. Since 2010, PHCRED-funded research has focused on:

● Improving access and reducing inequity.
● Better management of chronic conditions.

- Increasing the focus on prevention.
- Improving quality, safety, performance and accountability.[67]

Two organisations also funded under this strategy are the Australian Primary Health Care Research Institute (APHCRI), which commissions research, and the Primary Health Care Research and Information Service, which disseminates research.[67] In the first 10 years of PHCRED funding, 46 research grants, commissioned through APHCRI, focused primarily on health systems and services, while 116 grants, funded from the strategy but administered through the National Health and Medical Research Council (NHMRC), were more directed at clinical interventions.[68]

CURRENT ACTIVITY

Current research activity includes the nine APHCRI Centres of Research Excellence concentrating on chronic disease care in indigenous, rural and remote populations, transforming access to care, urban Aboriginal child health, primary oral healthcare, obesity management and prevention, the finance and economics of PHC, microsystem integration, and PHC care in rural and remote Australia. Uniquely, APHCRI has worked actively with these centres to enhance the adoption of their research into policy and practice.[69]

Examples of other significant primary care research include (but are not limited to) primary care cancer (Jon Emery), depression and multi-morbidity (Jane Gunn), dementia (Dimity Pond), cardiovascular disease prevention (Mark Nelson), prevention and its implementation (John Litt), management of HIV (Michael Kidd) and chronic disease management (Nick Zwar).

GAINS AND CHALLENGES

Two big challenges for primary care research are funding and research career pathways; nevertheless, progress is happening towards responding to both.

Through the NHMRC, the largest health and medical research funding body in Australia, less than 2% of grants awarded have been related to primary healthcare.[70] Nonetheless, primary care researchers are represented on NHMRC committees and faculties, and hence have an input on the management of this organisation.

Researchers have also attracted other funding from government, industry, professional bodies and philanthropic organisations. For example, the government-funded Bettering the Evaluation and Care of Health (BEACH) Program provides valued insights into what is happening in general practice, allowing us to measure the impact of changes in government policy and population health.[71]

FUTURE DIRECTIONS

While the PHC research workforce has been growing, it is hampered by the lack of formal training in PHC research methodologies, the scarcity of research funding and limited career opportunities. Addressing these issues, as well as providing mentoring and leadership development, would enable this workforce to become more productive and sustainable.[72] The recently announced Australian Academy of Health and Medical Sciences has been set up in part to focus on the development of future generations of health and medical researchers.[73]

Given the greater emphasis globally on primary care and prevention to improve health outcomes and a sustainable healthcare system, PHC research has the potential to play a significant role in achieving this.[74,75]

Promising opportunities lie with developing practice-based research networks supported by the national support service – the Australian Primary Care Research Network[76] – and the Primary Health Networks established to increase the efficiency and effectiveness of primary care services to ensure patients receive the right care in the right place at the right time.[77]

Increasing developments in research translation and utilisation, as seen in the formation of the NHMRC Research Translation Faculty,[78] and research-user willingness to engage more with researchers will see the acceleration of the transfer of research into policy and practice, leading to improvements in healthcare.

Africa Region

CHAPTER 38

Primary care research in South Africa

....

Gboyega Ogunbanjo and Bob Mash

HISTORY

Post-Apartheid South Africa has made the development of primary healthcare and provision of universal coverage a cornerstone of healthcare policy since 1994. This has redirected the attention of academic and higher education institutions towards a focus on family medicine and primary healthcare in both teaching and research. All nine health science faculties have departments of family medicine, and there has generally been increasing support for research that strengthens the country's commitment to primary healthcare.

Since the 1970s, South Africa has developed a model of vocational postgraduate training in family medicine that requires a research dissertation as part of a master's degree. This has necessitated a continuous group of trainees (now registrars) who are obligated to perform primary care research. At about the same time, the South African Academy of Family Practice and Primary Care (now the South African Academy of Family Physicians) developed a national journal – *South African Family Practice* – which has provided a regular opportunity to publish and share locally produced primary healthcare / family medicine research. The academy has also committed itself to annual National Family Practitioners conferences, with a strong emphasis on presentation and dissemination of research.

CURRENT ACTIVITY

Looking at the original research output published in *South African Family Practice* in 2014, one can see that the majority of primary care research has been either clinical or educational in nature. Clinical research was spread across the burden of disease with studies on HIV and TB, maternal and child health, non-communicable diseases as well as violence and trauma. The greatest activity has been on non-communicable diseases and the least activity on violence and trauma. However, there has been very little research on mental health. Educational research has focused on the development of the primary healthcare workforce and issues such as retention and recruitment in rural areas as well as the development of both under- and postgraduate education in family medicine. Very little activity has been seen in the areas of health services, health systems and the development of primary care research tools.

Methodologically, the emphasis remains on small-scale descriptive studies using surveys or qualitative interviews and quality improvement projects. Because the greatest activity is among registrars who perform a research assignment / dissertation as a part of their degree and clinical training, the topics and methods reflect the amount of time, expertise and funding available for such studies.

Family medicine remains the strongest academic discipline in primary healthcare, with much smaller contributions to the research output from primary healthcare nursing. Community health departments, the Medical Research Council and the Human Sciences Research Council have significant activity focused on health systems research, the burden of disease and national surveys such as the recently published South African National Health and Nutrition Examination Survey.[79]

GAINS AND CHALLENGES

Over the last few years, there has been an increasing emphasis on training at a doctoral level within the country. However, only two of the nine heads of department of family medicine hold a PhD. This limits the capacity for research supervision at a PhD level and the pursuit of larger scale and methodologically more ambitious projects that could benefit the primary healthcare system. Nevertheless, we are beginning to see a new group of more established researchers emerging and a growing community of PhD students in family medicine.

Funding for research within the South African context remains a challenge for everyone, and local bodies such as the Medical Research Council and National Research Foundation have historically only provided limited budgets for self-initiated research projects. The research agenda has been dominated and driven to a large extent by international funders who have focused on specific diseases such as HIV and TB as well as technological innovations. There has been very little funding available for the strengthening of health systems and services outside of specific disease-oriented programmes.

FUTURE DIRECTIONS

Over the next decade, we hope to see a substantial growth in the number of family physicians with doctorates. This will lead to a body of primary care research with more impact and contributions to the national policy on revitalising primary healthcare and ensuring universal coverage through the introduction of national health insurance. This should also improve the quality of supervision and research at both master's and PhD levels as well as creating a body of more established primary care researchers.

Although South Africa has a long way to go in terms of building primary care research capacity, we are beginning to share expertise and build research collaborations with other countries in sub-Saharan Africa. Networks such as Primary Care and Family Medicine Education (Primafamed; Africa) are focusing on research capacity building as one of their main tasks in the region and have also established the *African Journal of Primary Health Care & Family Medicine*. Collaborative multi-country research in the region offers exciting opportunities for larger-scale and relevant studies in the future.

CHAPTER 39

Primary care research in Kenya

· · · · · · · · · · · · · · · · · · · ·

Patrick Chege

HISTORY

The first Kenyan medical school (University of Nairobi) was established in Nairobi in 1967, and, as would be expected, the first documented medical research publications that involved Kenyan medical teachers followed within the next decade. The data provided by these publications were mainly on primary care.[80,81] These initial studies were conducted by internists and public health teachers as departments of family medicine and primary care were not established until four decades later. This medical school remained the only one until 1990, when the second medical school, Moi University School of Medicine, was established.

CURRENT ACTIVITY

It is notable that a large proportion of medical research conducted in Kenya continues to focus on primary care, although it is conducted by senior specialists in tertiary teaching hospitals.[82,83] The Moi University Department of Family Medicine admitted the first registrars in January 2005. The clinical training of these residents takes place in rural district/sub-district hospitals and rural faith-based hospitals. The Kenyan residency programmes in family medicine culminate in a master of medicine (MMed) degree. Most of the MMed research conducted by these residents in the last decade has been on patient management in these district health facilities. Levels of public health services in Kenya range from one to six, where one is in the community and six is the tertiary teaching hospital.[84] The faculty members of the Moi University Department of Family Medicine have engaged in district hospital- and community-based research in primary care.[85-88]

The most current primary care research activity involves chronic diseases and their complications (including HIV), fevers in children and reproductive health. The research work in these areas involves both clinicians and public health practitioners.

Research on health services delivery is starting to gain some momentum but is mostly in the hands of public health practitioners.

GAINS AND CHALLENGES

Research conducted in Kenya in primary care settings from the late 1960s until the 1990s was not acknowledged as primary care research. What is remarkable is the fact that it forms the foundation on which more specialised research has been conducted.[80-89]

The emphasis on research training in the family medicine residency programmes has stirred research interest, and the majority of the graduates (most of who are employees of the Ministry of Health [MOH]) are advocating for the MOH to support primary care research within the public health services (anecdotal data collected by author from discussions during local Kenyan conferences and workshops). This is unprecedented. With the growing focus on primary care by the World Health Organization and policymakers, primary care research is needed to inform both policymakers and primary care providers.[90]

The small number of well-trained research primary care team members in low-income countries such as Kenya makes the task of establishing and owning primary care research a challenging one.

FUTURE DIRECTIONS

The most promising opportunities for future primary care research in Kenya include:

1. The devolution of health services to fairly small political units (counties), which may enable more of focus on primary care and primary care research. Such research would focus on the quality and effectiveness of primary care and highlight areas that need improvement.
2. The growing interest in national health insurance among Kenyans, especially those that utilise the public health services. In Kenya, funds for the development of national health insurance are managed by the national government and more are now utilised at health facilities to improve services.
3. The proposed College of Family Physicians of East Africa is planned to enhance the training of private practitioners and accredit them as members or fellows to increase the number of providers that can be accredited to provide service under the national health insurance scheme.

CHAPTER 40

Primary care research in Ghana

....

Akye Essuman

HISTORY

The Danfa/Ghana comprehensive rural health and family planning project was conceptualised in 1964 and was one of the first opportunities for primary care research and development.[91] It was a collaboration involving the Ghana Medical School; the Ministry of Health; the University of California, Los Angeles; and the United States Agency for International Development (USAID). The aim was to demonstrate how successfully rural transformation can be achieved by communities themselves, aided by several agencies and institutions, under the leadership of health workers utilising existing resources more effectively. The objectives of the project were to investigate the state of the rural community, to train health workers, to provide a competent and well-oriented workforce to handle the problems of the community and to establish comprehensive and preventive health services through the Danfa Health Centre. To date, health students from the University of Ghana receive training in rural health from the Danfa group of villages.

The Community-Based Health Planning and Services (CHPS) concept began in 1999.[92] It was developed by the Navrongo Health Research Centre based on the 'Navrongo experiment' conducted in 1994. The CHPS 'zone' presently constitutes the basic unit of healthcare delivery in the Ghana Health Service and is managed by Community Health Officers.

The National Health Insurance Scheme (NHIS)[93] was launched in 2003, based on outcomes of previous research conducted in some districts in Ghana. The aim of the scheme was to ensure universal health insurance coverage and access to basic healthcare services for all residents in Ghana.

In another initiative, Ghana participated in multi-country research on ageing, health and well-being in older adults in 2007–2008.[94] Some significant findings were that women rated their health worse than men; in both sexes, health-related issues and old age were the main reasons for discontinuation of work; and there was a significant gap between self-reported diagnosis of hypertension (14%) and measured hypertension (55%) in older Ghanaians.

CURRENT ACTIVITY

A randomised trial of task-shifting and blood pressure control at the community level in Ghana is being conducted.[95] This study seeks to employ cost-effective strategy, task-shifting, to mitigate the rising cardiovascular disease epidemic in sub-Saharan African countries like Ghana. The study seeks to evaluate the implementation of the World Health Organization task-shifting strategy, making use of Ghana's already established community health worker programme, CHPS, integrated within the national health insurance scheme.

Another project is the scaling up of NHIS capitation to other regions in Ghana, after successfully piloting it in the Ashanti region of Ghana in 2013–2014.[96,97] Three additional regions are earmarked for inclusion by the end of 2015, to be followed by the remaining five regions by end of 2016.

Research is taking place on the impact of the rapid diagnostic test (RDT) in the management of malaria at the primary level.[98] It is expected that efficient application and interpretation of the RDT results will significantly reduce the presumptive treatment of febrile conditions such as malaria. The national malaria control programme requires providers to 'test, treat and track' suspected malaria cases.

Finally, the Ghana Ensure Mothers and Babies Regular Access to Care (EMBRACE) study was launched in 2012 jointly by the Japanese and Ghana governments.[99] The study aims to develop a pathway to create feasible and sustainable packages of interventions to improve maternal neonatal and child health outcomes, and to test such packages in rural settings. The intervention package includes continuum of care (COC) orientation for health workers, utilisation of a COC card, 24-hour retention at facility after delivery and a postnatal care home visit.

GAINS AND CHALLENGES

In terms of infrastructure, the Ministry of Health and the various universities have research centres strategically located in the northern, middle and southern belts of the country. Academic programmes in public health, family medicine and other primary care specialties that incorporate research are at different stages. Important achievements include improved healthcare delivery at the community level, reduction in maternal and infant mortality, reduction in prevalence of communicable diseases like HIV/AIDS and malaria, and eradication of communicable diseases like polio and guinea worm.

However, most clinicians are not involved in research for various reasons, such as having busy clinics, having inadequate training in research or simply not being interested. Primary care research is thus primarily left to public health physicians, who do comparatively little or no clinical work. Funding from local sources is virtually non-existent. External partners have funded most of the implementation research programmes.

FUTURE DIRECTIONS

Possible future projects include addressing implementation issues associated with scaling up the NHIS capitation system. Community-oriented primary care (COPC) as a component of the district health delivery system requires research. Through COPC, capacity will be built at the sub-district and community levels in addition to the provision of periodic specialised services at these lower centres. Other areas of research need are care of the elderly and hospice and palliative care.

CHAPTER 41

Primary care research in Nigeria

....

Olayinka Ayankogbe

HISTORY

Since 1980, when the first conference on training in family medicine (known then as general medical practice) was held in Nigeria, primary care research has been one of the issues targeted for academic development.[100]

Prior to this, medical research in Nigeria, even if it was primary care research, was not recognised as such, as primary care had not been defined within the Nigerian context, and the content of general medical practice/family medicine as a discipline was novel.

The commencement of the 4-year residency Fellowship Training Programme in Family Medicine in 1981, with a mandatory 2-year research project and writing of a research project dissertation, kick-started structured primary care research in Nigeria. The establishment of the *African Journal of Primary Health Care & Family Medicine* by the Primary Care and Family Medicine Education (Primafamed) Network, published in South Africa, also boosted primary care research in Nigeria to a great extent, as it provided an African platform for publication of regional research.

CURRENT ACTIVITY

Most research activities currently take place in the training institutions accredited for residency training in family medicine and are conducted by the residents. Clinical training settings include tertiary teaching hospitals, mission hospitals, federal medical centres, general hospitals and private general practices.

Larger-scale and significant research has been accomplished through research networks. An example of this is the mapping of reasons for patients seeking primary care in Nigerian primary care using the *International Classification of Primary Care*. Another ongoing interventional research project focuses on clinical training, where the medical directors of private general practices are taught transformational medical education methods in order to teach core family medicines skills to undergraduate medical students sent to them for a period of time.

GAINS AND CHALLENGES

The greatest primary care research capability in Nigeria lies in the units/departments of family medicine at the colleges of medicine/teaching hospitals scattered all over Nigeria, at both federal and state levels. Some of these departments have also established university-linked practice-based family medicine research networks, like the Family Medicine Unit at the College of Medicine, University of Lagos.

These research networks are also helping to establish links between general practitioners in practice and academic family physicians at university, with a collaborative focus on improving the quality of services rendered to the community.

The major challenge being faced is the resistance from other specialties to the growth of academic family medicine and the inability to understand the need for primary care research rather than just service delivery.

FUTURE DIRECTIONS

The most promising opportunities for building capability in, and increasing the amount of, primary care research lie in running academic university-based master's courses in family medicine. The Family Medicine Unit at the College of Medicine, University of Lagos, is planning to run a research-based postgraduate MSc course in family medicine by distance learning, and also hope to start running PhD courses in family medicine in the longer term.

It is intended that family medicine residents are encouraged to carry out practice-based research for their fellowship degree in family medicine, to strengthen the university-linked practice-based research network.

The Family Medicine Unit is also encouraging the residents and university lecturers to take the MPhil courses in family medicine run by the University of Stellenbosch in South Africa, to enhance their promotion in academia (ultimately to professors of family medicine).

Other opportunities include the intention to collaborate with family medicine networks in Africa (e.g. the Primafamed Network) and outside Africa (e.g. the North American Primary Care Research Group) to enhance primary care research. They also intend to continue to collaborate with the World Organization of Family Doctors Working Party on Research.

North America Region

CHAPTER 42

Primary care research in Canada

Gillian Bartlett and Jeannie Haggerty

HISTORY

Some of the key developments for primary care (PC) research in Canada can be traced back to the late 1960s in the first decades after the creation of the academic discipline of family medicine.[101] At this time, PC research was carried out principally by clinicians, usually without advanced training in research methods, and for whom research was the natural response to unanswered professional questions. Research productivity and complexity of methods increased dramatically, however, with the addition to family medicine departments of PhD scientists from a variety of disciplines in the early 2000s. A programme of PC research was built that was responsible for: (1) introducing one of the most highly cited frameworks for patient-centred medicine;[102,103] (2) providing evidence for the importance of moving from a single disease focus to multi-morbidity;[104,105] (3) establishing a method of participatory research that has promoted collaborative approaches to creating action-oriented knowledge, particularly in Aboriginal health;[106] and (4) building a research programme and methods to improve shared decision-making and knowledge translation in PC.[107]

CURRENT ACTIVITY

Based on the solid accomplishments of very active PC researchers, teams are now focusing on critical topics such as mental health, access for rural and remote populations, health of new immigrants and refugees and the burden of the ageing population with complex needs using community-based innovative approaches and engaging stakeholders in the research process. These topics are a reflection of the Canadian geographic and demographic characteristics that create specific challenges for the primary healthcare system. PC research in Canada tends to be grounded in the community in order to generate appropriate evidence for healthcare professional teams as well as patients and policymakers.

GAINS AND CHALLENGES

PC research capacity was catapulted forward as part of the massive investments in primary healthcare renewal between 2001 and 2006. This renewal engaged the community of PC researchers in evaluation efforts and led an unprecedented investment by the Canadian Institutes for Health Research (CIHR) in PC research and in the career support of mid-career researchers and of clinician-researchers. In addition, a major investment was made to create the Canadian Primary Care Sentinel Surveillance Network that receives electronic medical record data from PC clinics across the country, providing an invaluable research and quality assurance resource. These investments have drawn increased interest and improved the sustainability of PC research. These positive gains are offset by the fact that, in Canada, we actually have the equivalent of many different healthcare systems, as each province and the territories implement the Canada Health Care Act in different ways. These systems are spread over a very large geographical area for a relatively small population working with two official languages. Our greatest challenge at the moment is developing and sustaining meaningful research agendas in an overburdened, extremely complex, universal healthcare system with too few PC clinician scientists. As a result, we have lagged behind other comparable countries in our PC research outputs.[108]

FUTURE DIRECTIONS

There are several promising opportunities for PC research in Canada. First, Canada is taking the lead in developing and providing research training that is appropriate for PC. PC involves patient-oriented, community-based research that requires innovative methodologies and participatory approaches.[109,110] Programmes such as Transdisciplinary Understanding and Training of Research – Primary Health Care (TUTOR-PHC), a Canadian interdisciplinary inter-university fellowship and training programme that attracts the most promising PC research trainees, and new graduate programmes in family medicine at McGill University and Western University that train PC researchers with methods that build on different research traditions to address the complexities of PC while advancing academic excellence.

Second, the Primary Health Care Transition Fund in 2001–2005 invested C$800 million in renewal projects across Canada. One of the projects supported was the National Evaluation Strategy for PC that led to massive engagement of the research community to provide frameworks and methods. The Canadian Health Services Research Foundation started a PC network in 2005 to discuss how to capitalise on all the energy that was created and, especially, the close relationships developed between the PC research community and decision-makers and clinicians. The network com-missioned a report on the future of PC research. The report was a strong factor in the successful advocacy for our national funding agency (the CIHR) to invest in PC research capacity. Two influential groups were established: the Canadian Working Group on Primary Health Care Improvement and the Canadian Primary Care Research & Innovation Network.[111] This network is poised to be the coordinating centre for the Canadian Network on Primary and Integrated Health Care Innovations.

In addition, each province is establishing Support for People and Patient-Oriented Research and Trials (SUPPORT) units that are expected to be specialised resource centres. In Quebec, the decision was made to dedicate this unit to PC research.

All of these opportunities and support have really only occurred in the last 10 years. Our challenge will be to optimise the use of the resources provided and demonstrate benefit to the Canadian population and the primary healthcare system.

CHAPTER 43

Primary care research in the USA

. . . .

Larry Green

HISTORY

The development of formalised training of family physicians and of family medicine educational curricula in medical schools dominated family medicine enterprises during the 1960s and 1970s, crowding out attention to research until the 1980s. Then, fledgling efforts to develop the research workforce began to blossom through fellowships and direct mentoring of curious individuals. Concurrently, practice-based research networks (PBRNs) were invented and promulgated. Many local, regional and national PBRNs now exist and function as a foundational infrastructure for research using the full range of research methods for observational research, comparative effectiveness research, educational research, translational research and clinical trials.

During this period, consensus emerged that the knowledge base necessary for practising family medicine and serving people as personal physicians in the context of families and communities could not be discovered by other narrow fields of research and was an inescapable responsibility of family physicians and their colleagues. The great importance of embracing not only the biological and physical sciences but especially the behavioural sciences was exposed and fully accepted. Community-based participatory research emerged as a particularly relevant research method for family medicine. The gap between aspirations for use of digital personal health information and administrative data for research and what electronic health records could actually do was exposed and much effort devoted to closing it, with occasional success. Towards the end of this period, much attention turned to improving the platform for practice in the information age and linkage of primary care, public health and mental health to elevate individual and population health.

CURRENT ACTIVITY

Most family medicine and primary care researchers would identify as most salient what they are working on. Perhaps most would agree that health services research focused on developing the patient-centred medical home, its 'neighbourhood' and its proper financing are major foci of research activity. This area of engagement is aligned with the national policy goal of improving healthcare that actually improves individual and population health, affordably. This work can be thought of as modernising the primary care platform of healthcare delivery.

In response to several reports from the US Institute of Medicine, there is substantial research focused on integrating primary care with behavioural health (which includes substance use, unhealthy behaviours, mental health and other emotional difficulties). Basic research about extracting data from electronic records, linkage with population-level data from local and national surveys and stewarding these data for research purposes focused on particular localities is being enthusiastically pursued. This research about data acquisition and use, as never before possible, is linked to physician certification, quality improvement at the practice level, community engagement, education and training, and seems to be a key driver towards reuniting family medicine, primary care and public health.

GAINS AND CHALLENGES

Academic departments of family medicine and some academic divisions of general internal medicine and general paediatrics, combined with perhaps 150 PBRNs and a few large healthcare conglomerates, constitute the greatest primary care research capability. They are contributing to translational research that impacts patient-level decision-making (e.g. the Family Practice Inquiries Network) and redesigning practice models and improving the quality of frontline practice (e.g. chronic disease management, integrated care delivery).

A big challenge is confusion about roles in a chaotic aggregation of fragments of healthcare services, and another is the lack of a parsimonious, widely accepted set of measures that actually matter to patients and frontline clinicians – to guide improvement research. Data reporting requirements to an ever-increasing number of agencies, practice fatigue and an absence of capital for enhanced approaches to practice have united to create considerable scepticism about the future and drain professional motivation to ask and answer questions of importance to family physicians and their patients. The limitations of electronic health records remain a ubiquitous challenge for research.

FUTURE DIRECTIONS

There is probably no greater immediate opportunity for further primary care research than discovering how to reunite primary care, public health and behavioural health squarely focused on the goal of increased population health. This could be an antidote to the continuing march of the USA to the bottom of critical population health measures when compared with peer nations. Solving the data extraction–linkage–use equations and defining and agreeing on the family medicine / primary care data model and classification systems necessary for episode-epidemiology capable of discovering the origins of illness and disease and how health is won and lost – are longer term, hugely promising and important opportunities. Fanning the flames of educational research is also particularly enticing, given its neglect and seminal importance in producing the health professions workforce the population now needs but doesn't have. And, of course, there is the imminent opportunity to unite primary care with emerging genetic knowledge. Indeed, a splendid set of opportunities for the brightest and best.

Iberoamericana-CIMF* Region

CHAPTER 44

Primary care research in Uruguay

....

Jacqueline Ponzo

HISTORY

Historically, Uruguay had two significant periods of primary care research, during the 1960s and 1980s. Hugo Dibarboure Icasuriaga, a rural physician from the Florida Department, applied the scientific method to describe his community, the health service and the environment, as a resource and as feedback on his clinical practice.[112] Juan Carlos Macedo, from Migues, Canelones, also a rural area, led the Migues Medical Group that developed a model for longitudinal continuity in their primary care practice. The focus of clinical research was prevalent diseases in the elderly population from the area and the study provided evidence to defend the quality of primary care.[113] The main works were only published in the *Medical Journal of Uruguay* after 1985, when the military dictatorship (1973–1985) that had a very negative impact on the academic life of the country, had ended. The *Medical Journal of Uruguay* had been seized by the military government during this time. Besides these cases, research in the area of health in Uruguay in these years was focused on basic and clinical research, particularly gynaecology and obstetrics.

Rebuilding the country after the period of authoritarianism was a slow process. Research was not a priority, and the start of family and community medicine residency

---

* Confederación Iberoamericana de la Medicina Familiar (Latin American Confederation of Family Medicine).

in 1997 was the beginning of a new era that is slowly consolidating primary care with an academic perspective in which research is gradually emerging as a natural activity linked to its pioneers.

CURRENT ACTIVITY

Since 2008, health reform has emphasised primary healthcare with an orientation towards family and community. Later in that year, with the participation of specialists in family and community medicine, public health and social sciences, the Primary Care Assessment Tool Uruguay (PCAT.UY) group was formed as a research group within the University of the Republic with the goal of contributing to the assessment of the new model of primary care. Initial work was performed in collaboration with other researchers in the region from Brazil, Spain and Argentina[114] as well as Barbara Starfield, who developed the original Primary Care Assessment Tool in the USA.[115] From 2009 to 2013 research on PCAT was carried out and the PCAT Provider and PCAT Adults consumer versions (the UR-PCAT PE and UR-PCAT AE, respectively) were developed and adapted for Uruguay.[116] In 2010, Barbara Starfield visited Montevideo, where the first meeting of PCAT researchers from the region took place and which would later evolve into what is now the Ibero America PCAT Collaboration, with an important contribution from Uruguay.[117] Although lack of funding has prevented the widespread application of the instrument, collaboration has developed with PCAT groups that have emerged in other countries such as Ecuador, Colombia, Bolivia and Mexico.[118]

In 2009, Uruguay was part of the team that received funding from the US National Institutes of Health for the Center of Excellence for Cardiovascular Health in South America (CESCAS) Project, a longitudinal study of risk factors and cardiovascular and respiratory disease in the Southern Cone.[119] The Uruguayan focus in this project is on research tools to track participants and on the training of researchers.

A new curriculum for undergraduate medical training in Uruguay was developed in 2009, which prioritises training in research methodology. During 2014, the first compulsory practical experience was undertaken, which resulted in monographs, some of which are in primary care.

GAINS AND CHALLENGES

The main achievements Uruguay has made are a basic infrastructure, generated through participation in the previously mentioned projects, a collaborative scenario at regional and sub-regional levels, and the development of young researchers with theoretical and practical training.

The main challenges are to achieve continuity and to deepen what has been achieved. More determined policies and better financial support for research in primary care are needed.

FUTURE DIRECTIONS

Future primary care research should focus on topics derived from current unsolved health problems and needs and utilise the emerging expertise in research. Such topics include the complexity of the problems of violence and drug abuse, the treatment of chronic diseases and multi-morbidity, the non-specific mental problems that arise along with other health problems, the management of primary care services and the assessment of health system reforms.

Interdisciplinary work and the integration of different techniques and methodologies are necessary when it comes to research questions that go beyond biomedical topics. Collaboration with the humanities, social scientists and environmental professionals is needed.

Continuity in the training of young students to pursue research-oriented master's and doctoral degrees is the next step that will allow the consolidation of teams for the development of the necessary research.

CHAPTER 45

Primary care research in Mexico

....

José Ramirez Aranda

HISTORY

Beginning in 1990, one of the most important developments in primary care research in Mexico was the creation of three specialised journals of family medicine: *Archivos de Medicina Familiar* (1999–2010), which is now inactive; *Atención Familiar* (2004), the official publication of the Universidad Nacional Autónoma de México (UNAM); and the *Revista Mexicana de Medicina Familiar* (2014), the official publication of the Mexican College of Family Medicine (CMMF).[120]

In the same way, since 1988, annual national congresses of family medicine, as forums for the exchange of ideas, and less frequently, colloquia of research professor associations, are held.[121] In 2006, a virtual network of Latin American research professors was started; unfortunately, it disappeared in 2011.[122] In 2010, the Researchers Network of the Mexican College of Family Medicine was started with the participation of 11 states of the Mexican Republic, with tangible achievements in scientific productivity and with the participation of other research groups.

CURRENT ACTIVITY

Primary care research is mainly conducted in public academic institutions such as the institutes and schools of public health of Morelos, Veracruz, and Nuevo León, among others and in health science schools in universities in several cities in Mexico. In the specific area of family medicine, the Institute of Mexican Social Security (IMSS), the home of family medicine residency training, carries out research, as do university departments of family medicine (i.e. UNAM, Universidad Autónoma de Nuevo León, Universidad de Guadalajara, Universidad Autónoma de San Luis Potosí Inicio and others).

However, within such public institutions, primary care research makes up only a small percentage of the research output. For example, primary care research makes up only 3% of the output from the Institute for Social Security and Services for State

Workers and 16% of that from the IMSS.[123] Only 10% of the members of the state association of family medicine publish.[124] The recently formed Researchers Network of the CMMF has a relevant role with regard to the generation and dissemination of primary care research.

In general, primary care research activities in Mexico are insufficient in relation to the significance of the discipline in the academic setting, and 90% of the work is descriptive with little impact on the discipline of family medicine or other specialties.

GAINS AND CHALLENGES

Public academic institutions and university departments perform research focused on clinical practice; however, in the institution representative of family medicine, the IMSS, the practice of family medicine is largely focused on clinical activities. It has, however, succeeded in maintaining a primary care journal since 1969, which includes clinical and public health research.[125]

The university departments of family medicine encourage research in their teaching and require research studies in order to obtain the degree of family medicine; unfortunately, few are published. The establishment of a research network in family medicine with international cooperation with the North American Primary Care Research Group (NAPCRG) and the Ibero-American Research Network in Family Medicine (IBIMEFA) is promising. One of the greatest challenges is the development of human resources in research who will exercise greater scientific rigor, increase scientific productivity, achieve greater consistency in findings, and provide more credibility to the discipline.[126]

Other challenges are the development of competency in qualitative research, having professional researchers tutor primary care physicians, the creation of strategic alliances to nurture primary care[127] and, fundamentally, identifying sources of research funding.

FUTURE DIRECTIONS

The organisation of research networks through synchronous or real-time communication seems to be the answer to the need for effective communication between researchers, for distance tutoring, to carry out multicentre studies and to achieve greater standing for the specialty.

The creation of a family medicine journal as a means of dissemination for the Mexican College of Family Medicine will fulfil an urgent need for transmitting generated knowledge; this is needed because the previous two journals are no longer in circulation.

Cooperation with international research groups such as the NAPCRG, the IBIMEFA, and the International Implementation Research Network in Primary Care, represent a great opportunity for the growth and development of primary care research in Mexico. Primary care research must respond to the needs of medical practice and focus on understanding aspects of human illness, uncertainty, prevention and patient-centred care in our context. For this, qualitative research holds an important position.

CHAPTER 46

Primary care research in Brazil

. . . .

Magda Almeida, Gustavo Gusso and Thiago Trindade

HISTORY

The first Brazilian article on primary healthcare (PHC) dates back to 1977[128] and deals with the need to reorganise the outpatient services model in a university hospital. It highlighted the effectiveness of PHC features and the importance of training human resources in this practice scenario.

The organisation of PHC in Brazil began officially in 1994, with the implementation of the Family Health Program, which created posts for family doctors. In turn, this created a career path, a need for specialised training and a demand for more research. Parallel to this, the Brazilian Society of Family and Community Medicine (SBMFC) started to organise scientific meetings, and many health workers wanted to present posters and started to perform 'simple' research projects such as cross-sectional studies and case reports.

Although the first issue of the *Brazilian Journal of Family and Community Medicine* was published in 1987, it subsequently stopped publishing and was only reactivated in 2004. In 2010, the Primary Health Care Research Network was established to provide better communication and coordination between Brazilian PHC researchers, practitioners, users and managers, and to promote better use of research results within PHC. This network is funded by the Primary Health Care Department of the Ministry of Health and is operated and developed by the Brazilian Association of Graduate Studies in Public Health, with national and international partner and sponsor institutions.

Subsequently, there was a significant increase in the number of Brazilian articles published with 'primary health care' and 'primary care' descriptors. In 2014 alone, 214 articles used these descriptors. In total for the 26 years, there were 965 PHC-related articles in the Scientific Electronic Library Online (SciELO) database, of which 96% were published after 1998. In the Latin American and Caribbean Health Sciences Literature (LILACS) database, there are even more publications, with 1368 Brazilian articles on PHC, 70% of which were published after 2008.

Many articles are in Portuguese and not in indexed journals. When searching Google Scholar for the term 'primary healthcare' in Portuguese, from 1970 to 2000, there were 1370 articles, and, from 2001 to 2015, an increase to 19 000 results, which demonstrates the development of interest in primary care research. A search of PubMed returned 193 articles in Portuguese from 1970 to 2000 and 993 from 2001 to 2015. These are not only Brazilian articles, and probably reflect the growth of primary care research worldwide, not only in Brazil.

CURRENT ACTIVITY

In Brazil, health sciences, humanities and applied social sciences are the major contributors to primary care research. Public, environmental and occupational health are the subject areas with the greatest number of published works, and the professional category of nursing is the one with most studies on PHC.

The main research questions in Brazil have been 'Is the Brazilian public health system effective?' and 'What is the best model to organise primary care?' This focus has resulted in many ecological or observational studies being published. Many projects also focused on community health workers (health community agents), who were central to the Family Health Programme. Many studies have been of low quality and illustrate a 'Rosenthal effect',[129] which means that the opinion of the main researcher had a great influence on the methods and results. Something similar occurred with researchers who tried to prove that group activities inside health centres were effective using qualitative studies. Another bias in the historical Brazilian scientific production in public health is the focus on 'programmes', such as those concerning children's health, women's health and chronic diseases. These biases are shown in a relevant series published in *The Lancet*.[130,131]

A range of new research policies and training courses have contributed to increased research on the training of human resources for PHC. These studies have focused on undergraduate training, postgraduate training at a master's level as well as programmes such as the Work Education Program for Health (PET-Saúde), which integrates education and service in the community.

The evaluation of public health policies has been constantly fostered by the possibility of financing research projects through public funding agencies, which systematically launch tenders for large national and state competition.

GAINS AND CHALLENGES

Clinical disease-related programme assessment have been targeted by various public policies. The production of PHC research in Brazil can be understood as a reflection of this political priority, since it has followed the trend of analysing and evaluating health services and work processes.

Clinical research on PHC is still incipient in the country, both with regard to the prevention and early diagnosis of diseases and the monitoring and managing of chronic illnesses. Nationally, most PHC research remains descriptive (case reports and prevalence studies), and analytical or experimental studies are rare. The main analytical work occurs through the analysis of routinely collected health indicators.

The focus has been changing from a big macro level to an intermediate level. Research about the organisation of primary care at the health centre level has increased. The SBMFC and the Ministry of Health have published many books and tools that have helped this research growth. The most important of these have been the translation of the *International Classification of Primary Care* (ICPC),[132] the validation of a national list of Ambulatory Care Sensitive Conditions and the translation and validation of the Primary Care Assessment Tool (PCAT).[133] The presence of Professor Barbara Starfield from 2000 to 2010 in many scientific meetings was very important to encourage health professionals and researchers to find a focus.

FUTURE DIRECTIONS

The national PHC computerisation project (E-SUS Atenção Básica) should enable collation and analysis of clinical and pharmaceutical data at the federal and municipal levels. If used properly, this tool has the potential to yield important information on Brazilian PHC patients.

It is necessary to invest in the production of new lightweight technologies to deal with mental diseases and for the control of cardio-metabolic diseases that affect a large portion of people seeking PHC services. We need to urgently balance the culture of predominantly health services and systems–oriented research with clinical research that addresses the local burden of disease and guides clinical practice.

SECTION V REFERENCES

1. Howie JG, Whitfield M, editors. *Academic General Practice in the UK Medical Schools, 1948–2000: A Short History.* Edinburgh: Edinburgh University Press, 2011.

2. Society for Academic Primary Care (SAPC). *New Century, New Challenges: A Report from the Heads of Departments of General Practice and Primary Care in the Medical Schools of the United Kingdom.* London: SAPC, 2002.

3. Medical Research Council (MRC). *MRC Topic Review: Primary Health Care.* London: MRC, 1997.

4. Mant D. *R&D in Primary Care: National Working Group Report.* London: Department of Health, 1997. Available at: http://webarchive.nationalarchives.gov.uk/20130107105354/http://www.dh.gov.uk/prod_consum_dh/idcplg?IdcService=GET_FILE&dID=2158&Rendition=Web (accessed 29 November 2015).

5. National Health Service (NHS) National Institute for Health Research (NIHR). Funding. Available at: http://www.nihr.ac.uk/funding/ (accessed 30 November 2015).

6. NHS NIHR. School for Primary Care Research. Available at: http://www.nihr.ac.uk/funding/school-for-primary-care-research.htm (accessed 30 November 2015).

7. Little P, chief investigator; University of Southampton, contractor. Positive Online WEight Reduction (POWER) [trial]. Project identifier: HTA – 09/127/19. Available at: http://www.nets.nihr.ac.uk/projects/hta/0912719 (accessed 30 November 2015).

8. Gilbody S, chief investigator; The University of York, contractor. The CASPER-PLUS Trial: Collaborative care for screen-positive elders with Major Depressive Disorder. Project identifier: HTA – 10/57/43. Available at: http://www.nets.nihr.ac.uk/projects/hta/105743 (accessed 30 November 2015).

9. Moore M, Yuen HM, Dunn N et al. Explaining the rise in antidepressant prescribing: a descriptive study using the general practice research database. *BMJ* 2009; **339**: b3999. [Erratum appears in *BMJ* 2009; **339**: b4361.]

10. Osborn DP, Baio G, Walters K et al. Inequalities in the provision of cardiovascular screening to people with severe mental illnesses in primary care: cohort study in the United Kingdom THIN Primary Care Database 2000–2007. *Schizophrenia Research* 2011; **129**(2–3): 104–10.

11. Yardley L, chief investigator; Solent NHS Trust, contractor. Integrating Digital Interventions into Patient Self-Management Support (DIPSS). Project identifier: RP-PG-1211-20001. Available at: http://www.nihr.ac.uk/funding/funded-research/funded-research.htm?postid=2251 (accessed 30 November 2015).

12. Lewis G, chief investigator; University of Bristol, contractor. PANDA: What are the indications for prescribing antidepressants that will lead to a clinical benefit? Project identifier: 13090. Available at: http://public.ukcrn.org.uk/search/StudyDetail.aspx?StudyID=13090 (accessed 30 November 2015).

13. Little P, Stuart B, Francis N et al. Effects of internet-based training on antibiotic prescribing rates for acute respiratory-tract infections: a multinational, cluster, randomised, factorial, controlled trial. *Lancet* 2013; **382**(9899): 1175–82.

14. Inskip HM, Dunn N, Godfrey KM et al. Is birth weight associated with risk of depressive symptoms in young women? Evidence from the Southampton Women's Survey. *American Journal of Epidemiology* 2008; **167**(2): 164–8.

15. Vedsted P, Olesen F. A differentiated approach to referrals from general practice to support early cancer diagnosis – the Danish three-legged strategy. *British Journal of Cancer* 2015; **112** (Suppl. 1): S65–9.

16. Segura-Fragoso A, Segura-Rodríguez A. Revisión de los estudios sobre producción científica de Atención Primaria publicados en España desde 1985 a 2008 [Review of the bibliometric

studies on primary care scientific production published in Spain from 1985 to 2008] [Spanish]. *Semergen* 2010; **36**(2): 75–81.

17. López-Torres Hidalgo J, Basora Gallisà J, Orozco Beltrán D et al. Mapa bibliométrico de la investigación realizada en atención primaria en España durante el periodo 2008–2012 [Bibliometric map of research done in primary care in Spain during the period 2008–2012] [Spanish]. *Atención Primaria* 2014; **46**(10): 541–8.

18. Violán Fors C, GrandesOdriozola G, Zabaleta-del-Olmo E et al. La investigación en atención primaria como área de conocimiento. Informe SESPAS 2012 [Research in primary care as an area of knowledge: SESPAS Report 2012] [Spanish]. *Gaceta Sanitaria* 2012; **26** (Suppl. 1): 76–81.

19. Bellón JÁ, Lopez-Tórres J. La investigación en Atención Primaria como área de conocimiento [Research in primary care as knowledge area] [Spanish]. *Atención Primaria* 2012; **44**(4): 185–6.

20. Heath I. Overdiagnosis: when good intentions meet vested interests; an essay by Iona Heath. *BMJ* 2013; **347**: f6361.

21. Ünlüoğlu İ. Academic promotions in the discipline of family medicine and oral exams for associate professorship. *Turkish Journal of Family Practice* 2013; **17**(3): 137–41.

22. Güldal D, Başak O. Twenty years of academic family medicine departments in Turkey: an overview on the developmental process. *Turkish Journal of Family Practice* 2014; **18**(1): 16–24.

23. Kringos D, Boerma W, Bourgueil Y et al. The strength of primary care in Europe: an international comparative study. *British Journal of General Practice* 2013; **63**(616): e742–50.

24. Akman M. Strength of primary care in Turkey. *Turkish Journal of Family Practice* 2014; **18**(2): 72–8.

25. Akman M, Kalaça S, Sargın M. QUALICOPC: a multi-country study evaluating quality, costs and equity in primary care. *Turkish Journal of Family Practice* 2012; **16**(2): 68–71.

26. Hummers-Pradier E, Beyer M, Chevallier P. *Research Agenda for General Practice / Family Medicine and Primary Health Care in Europe*. Maastricht: European General Practice Research Network (EGPRN), 2009. Available at: http://www.egprn.org/files/userfiles/file/research_agenda_for_general_practice_family_medicine.pdf (accessed 29 November 2015).

27. Polliack MR, Medalie JH. Programme for specialization in family medicine. *British Medical Journal* 1969; **4**(5681): 487–9.

28. Medalie JH, Levene C, Papier C et al. Blood groups, myocardial infarction and angina pectoris among 10,000 adult males. *New England Journal of Medicine* 1971; **285**(24): 1348–53.

29. Doron H, Shvartz S, Vinker S. [*Family Medicine in Israel: Its Origins, History and Significance in the Israeli Health Care System*] [Hebrew]. The Negev: Ben-Gurion University, 2015.

30. Borkan J, Van Tulder M, Reis S et al. Advances in the field of low back pain in primary care: a report from the fourth international forum. *Spine* 2002; **27**(5): E128–32.

31. Cohen Castel O, Keinan-Boker L, Geyer O et al. Factors associated with adherence to glaucoma pharmacotherapy in the primary care setting. *Family Practice* 2014; **31**(4): 453–61.

32. Gordon B, Afek A, Livshits S et al. The association between body mass index and increased utilization of healthcare services: a retrospective cohort study of 51,521 young adult males. *Endocrine Practice* 2014; **20**(7): 638–45.

33. Goldfracht M, Levin D, Peled O et al. Twelve-year follow-up of a population-based primary care diabetes program in Israel. *International Journal for Quality in Health Care* 2011; **23**(6): 674–81.

34. Ayalon L, Karkabi K, Bleichman I et al. Between modern and traditional values: Informal mental health help-seeking attitudes according to Israeli Arab women, primary care patients and their providers. *International Journal of Social Psychiatry* 2015; **61**(4): 386–93.

35. Shvartzman P, Singer Y, Bentur N et al. Constructing a post-graduate palliative care curriculum: the Israeli National Palliative Care Training (INPACT) experience. *Journal of Palliative Care* 2011; **27**(3): 238–43.

36. Minerbi A, Vulfsons S. Pain medicine in crisis: a possible model toward a solution; empowering community medicine to treat chronic pain. *Rambam Maimonides Medical Journal* 2013; **4**(4): e0027.

37. Alnasir F. Family medicine in the Arab world? Is it a luxury? *Journal Bahrain Medica Society*, Jan–Mar 2009: **21**(1): 191–2. Available at www.moh.gov.bh/EN/MOHServices/Services/primaryHealthCare.aspx (accessed 5 February 2016).

38. Hunt V. Bahrain's Family medicine residency program. *Bahrain Medical Bulletin* 1981; **3**(2): 60–8.

39. Alnasir F. The Watched Structured Clinical Examination (WASCE) as a tool of assessment. *Saudi Medical Journal* 2004; **25**(1): 71–4.

40. Al-Nasir FA, Robertson AS. Can selection assessments predict students' achievements in the premedical year? A study at Arabian Gulf University. *Education for Health* 2001; **14**(2): 277–86.

41. Alnasir F, Jaradat A. Prediction of medical students' performance in the medical school. *Family Medicine & Medical Science Research* 2013; **2**: 113.

42. Kingdom of Bahrain Ministry of Health (MOH) Family Practice Residency Program (FPRP). Teaching activities. Available at: http://familymedicine.moh.gov.bh/TeachingActivities.aspx (accessed 30 November 2015).

43. Kingdom of Bahrain MOH FPRP. Research and publications. Available at: http://familymedicine.moh.gov.bh/ResidentsResearch.aspx (accessed 30 November 2015).

44. Al-Jalahma M, Fakhroo E. Teaching medical ethics: implementation and evaluation of a new course during residency training in Bahrain. *Education for Health* 2004; **17**(1): 62–72.

45. Al Khaja KA, Sequeira RP, Al-Ansari TM et al. Prescription writing skills of residents in a family practice residency programme in Bahrain. *Postgraduate Medical Journal* 2008; **84**(990): 198–204.

46. [Application form for 2013 *Bahrain Medical Bulletin* research fund.] Bahrain: Research Committee of the *Bahrain Medical Bulletin*, 2013. Available at: www.bahrainmedicalbulletin.com/Checklist_Application (accessed 27 November 2015).

47. Dandona L, Raban MZ, Guggilla RK et al. Trends of public health research output from India during 2001–2008. *BMC Medicine* 2009; **7**: 59.

48. Ministry of Health. *National Health Policy 2002*. Available at: www.mohfw.nic.in/showfile.php?lid=2325 (accessed 5 February 2016).

49. Solomon SS, Tom SC, Pichert J et al. Impact of medical student research in the development of physician-scientists. *Journal of Investigative Medicine* 2003; **51**(3): 149–56.

50. Mehra SJ. Spice route movement: forum for young and future family physicians / primary care physicians of South Asia. *Journal of Family Medicine and Primary Care* 2012; **1**(1): 62–5.

51. Ejaz K, Shamim MS, Shamim MS et al. Involvement of medical students and fresh medical graduates of Karachi, Pakistan in research. *Journal of Pakistan Medical Association* 2011; **61**(2): 115–20.

52. Aslam F, Shakir M, Qayyum MA. Why medical students are crucial to the future of research in South Asia. *PLoS Medicine* 2005; **2**(11): e322.

53. Kannan K, Thankappan K, Ramankutty V, Aravindan K. Kerala: a unique model of development. *Health Millions* 1991 Dec; **17**(5): 30–3.

54. Weiyuan C. China's village doctors take great strides. *Bulletin of the World Health Organization* 2008; **86**(12): 914–15.

55. Institute of Medicine. *A Manpower Policy for Primary Health Care: Report of a Study.* Washington DC: National Academy of Sciences, 1978.

56. Ministry of Health (MOH) Malaysia. MOH History. Available at: http://www.moh.gov.my/ english.php/pages/view/532 (accessed 29 November 2015).

57. MOH Malaysia Disease Control Division Non-Communicable Disease Section. *National Strategic Plan for Non-Communicable Disease (NSPNCD): Medium Term Strategic Plan to Further Strengthen the Cardiovascular Diseases and Diabetes Prevention and Control Program in Malaysia.* Putrajaya: MOH Malaysia Disease Control Division Non-Communicable Disease Section, 2010.

58. Khoo E, Teng C, Ng C et al. *Bibliography of Primary Care Research in Malaysia.* Kuala Lumpur: University Malaya Press, 2008.

59. Ministry of Health, Malaysia. Family medicine services. *Malaysia's Health 2002: Technical Report of the Director-General of Health, Malaysia.* Putrajaya: MOH Malaysia Family Health Division, 2002.

60. MOH Malaysia. *Annual Report 2012.* MOH/S/RAN/55.13(AR). Putrajaya: MOH Malaysia, 2012. Available at: http://vlib.moh.gov.my/cms/documentstorage/com.tms.cms.document. Document_433472a1-a02c4149-1b47cc20-e49f321e/2012%20%28English%29.pdf (accessed 29 November 2015).

61. Academy of Medicine Malaysia. Clinical Practice Guidelines. Available at: http://www. acadmed.org.my/index.cfm?&menuid=67 (accessed 29 November 2015).

62. Malaysian Primary Care Research Group (MPCRG) [homepage]. Available at: mpcrg.net (accessed 29 November 2015).

63. Academy of Family Physicians of Malaysia [homepage]. Available at: http://elms.afpm.org. my/portal/ (accessed 30 November 2015).

64. Lawson KA, Chew M, Van der Weyden MB. The rise and rise of academic general practice in Australia. *Medical Journal of Australia* 1999; **171**(11–12): 643–8.

65. Raupach JC, Pilotto LS. Randomised trials within the general practice evaluation program. Why so few? *Australian Family Physician* 2001; **30**(5): 504–7.

66. Australian Government Department of Health and Ageing. *Primary Health Care Research, Evaluation and Development (PHCRED) Strategy: Phase Three: 2010–2014.* Canberra: Australian Government Department of Health and Ageing, 2010. Available at: http://www. health.gov.au/internet/main/publishing.nsf/Content/02DB30DFFAC002E8CA257BF0001C FF3C/$File/PHCRED%20Strategy%20Oct%202010%20PRINT.pdf (accessed 29 November 2015).

67. Brown LJ, McIntyre EL. The contribution of Primary Health Care Research, Evaluation and Development-supported research to primary health care policy and practice. *Australian Journal of Primary Health* 2014; **20**(1): 47–55.

68. Yen L, Kalucy L, Ward N et al. *Stocktake of Primary Health Care Research in Australia.* Australian Primary Health Care Research Institute and Primary Health Care Research and Information Service, 2010. Available at: http://www.phcris.org.au/phplib/filedownload. php?file=/elib/lib/downloaded_files/publications/pdfs/phcris_pub_8381.pdf (accessed 29 November 2015).

69. Australian Primary Health Care Research Institute. Centres of Research Excellence. Available at: http://aphcri.anu.edu.au/aphcri-network/centres-research-excellence-cres (accessed 30 November 2015).

70. McIntyre EL, Mazza D, Harris NP. NHMRC funding for primary health care research, 2000–2008. *Medical Journal of Australia* 2011; **195**(4): 230.

71. Family Medicine Research Centre. Bettering the Evaluation and Care of Health (BEACH). Available at: http://sydney.edu.au/medicine/fmrc/beach/index.php (accessed 30 November 2015).

72. Oliver-Baxter J, Brown L, Yen L. Building the primary health care research workforce in Australia. 2015. http://aphcri.anu.edu.au/whats-on/all-news/primary-health-care-research-workforce-project.

73. Australian Academy of Health and Medical Sciences [homepage]. Available at: www.aahms.org (accessed 30 November 2015).

74. Russell LM. *Primary Care and General Practice in Australia 1990–2012: A Chronology of Federal Government Strategies, Policies, Programs and Funding.* Acton: Australian National University, 2013. Available at: http://aphcri.anu.edu.au//files/primary_care_and_general_practice_update_may_2013.pdf (accessed 29 November 2015).

75. Australian Government Productivity Commission. Efficiency in Health: Productivity Research Paper. Canberra: Australian Government Productivity Commission, 2015. Available at: http://www.pc.gov.au/research/completed/efficiency-health/efficiency-health.pdf (accessed 29 November 2015).

76. Australian Primary Care Research Network [homepage]. Available at: www.apcren.org.au (accessed 30 November 2015).

77. Australian Government Department of Health. Primary Health Networks (PHNs). Available at: www.health.gov.au/internet/main/publishing.nsf/content/primary_health_networks (accessed 30 November 2015).

78. Australian Government National Health and Medical Research Council. Research Translation Faculty. Available at: www.nhmrc.gov.au/research/research-translation/research-translation-faculty (accessed 30 November 2015).

79. Shisana O, Labadarios D, Rehle T et al.; SANHANES-1 Team. *South African National Health and Nutrition Examination Survey (SANHANES-1).* Cape Town: HSRC Press, 2013. Available at: http://www.hsrc.ac.za/uploads/pageNews/72/SANHANES-launch%20edition%20%28online%20version%29.pdf (accessed 29 November 2015).

80. Arya OP, Bennett FJ. Role of the medical auxiliary in the control of sexually transmitted disease in a developing country. *British Journal of Venereal Disease* 1976; **52**(2): 116–21.

81. Dissevelt AG, Kornman JJ, Vogel LC. An antenatal record for identification of high risk cases by auxiliary midwives at rural health centres. *Tropical and Geographical Medicine* 1976; **28**(3): 251–5.

82. Owiti PO, Owuor K, Ng'eno H et al. Characteristics of clients undergoing repeat HIV counseling and testing compared to clients newly tested for HIV in Nyanza Province, Kenya. *AIDS Research and Human Retroviruses* 2014; **30**(Suppl. 1): A216.

83. Vreeman RC, Nyandiko WM, Liu H et al. Measuring adherence to antiretroviral therapy in children and adolescents in western Kenya. *Journal of the International AIDS Society* 2014; **17**: 19227.

84. Ministry of Medical Services, Ministry of Public Health and Sanitation. *Kenya Health Policy 2012–2030.* Nairobi: Ministry of Medical Services and Ministry of Public Health and Sanitation, 2012. Available at: http://countryoffice.unfpa.org/kenya/drive/FinalKenyaHealthPolicyBook.pdf (accessed 29 November 2015).

85. Bloomfield GS, Mwangi A, Chege P et al. Multiple cardiovascular risk factors in Kenya: evidence from a health and demographic surveillance system using the WHO STEPwise approach to chronic disease risk factor surveillance. *Heart* 2013; **99**(18): 1323–9.

86. Kirui NK, Pastakia S, Kamano JH et al. Important co-morbidity in patients with diabetes mellitus in three clinics in Western Kenya. *Public Health Action* 2012; **2**(4): 148–51.

87. O'Meara W, Laktabai J, Armstrong J et al. Clinical characteristics of pediatric fevers in Western Kenya. Poster abstract presented at IDWeek: Advancing Science, Improving Care, San Francisco, 5–6 October 2013.

88. Obala AA, Simiyu CJ, Odhiambo DO et al. Webuye Health and Demographic Surveillance Systems baseline survey of soil-transmitted helminths and intestinal protozoa among children up to five years. *Journal of Tropical Medicine* 2013; **2013**: 734562.

89. Darragh JH, Hutchinson AR, Mngola EN. The diabetic clinic, Kenyatta National Hospital: review of results of treatment, and recommendations. *East African Medical Journal* 1971; **48**(7): 327–35.

90. Chan M. The rising importance of family medicine. Keynote address at the 2013 World Congress of the World Organization of Family Doctors, Prague, Czech Republic, 26 June 2013. Available at: http://www.who.int/dg/speeches/2013/family_medicine_20130626/en/ (accessed 29 November 2015).

91. Sai F, Wurapa F, Quartey-Papafio E. The Danfa/Ghana comprehensive rural health and family planning project: a community approach. *Ghana Medical Journal* 1972; **11**(1): 9–17.

92. Nyonator FK, Awoonor-Williams JK, Phillips JF et al. The Ghana Community-Based Health Planning and Services Initiative for scaling up service delivery innovation. *Health Policy and Planning* 2005; **20**(1): 25–34.

93. Blanchet NJ, Fink G, Osei-Akoto I. The effect of Ghana's National Health Insurance Scheme on health care utilisation. *Ghana Medical Journal* 2012; **46**(2): 76–84.

94. Biritwum R, Mensah G, Yawson A et al. *Ghana: Study on Global AGEing and Adult Health (SAGE) Wave 1*. Geneva: World Health Organization (WHO), 2013.

95. Ogedegbe G, Plange-Rhule J, Gyamfi J et al. A cluster-randomized trial of task shifting and blood pressure control in Ghana: study protocol. *Implementation Science* 2014; **9**: 73.

96. Opoku N, Nsiah R, Oppong P et al. *The Effect of Capitation Payment on the National Health Insurance Scheme in Ashanti Region, Ghana*. 2014. Available at: http://dx.doi.org/10.2139/ssrn.2479305 (accessed 29 November 2015).

97. Mensah SA. *Presentation at Health Partner's Summit (MOH)*. GIMPA. Accra: Ghana Institute of Management and Public Administration (GIMPA), 2015. Available at: http://moh-ghana.org/UserFiles/2015Summit/NHIS.pdf (accessed 27 November 2015).

98. Ansah EK, Narh-Bana S, Affran-Bonful H et al. The impact of providing rapid diagnostic malaria tests on fever management in the private retail sector in Ghana: a cluster randomized trial. *BMJ* 2015; **350**: h1019.

99. Ghana Ensure Mothers and Babies Regular Access to Care (EMBRACE) Implementation Research Team. *Ghana EMBRACE Implementation Research*. Accra: GIMPA, 2015. Available at: http://moh-ghana.org/UserFiles/2015Summit/EMBRACE%20presentation.pdf (accessed 27 November 2015).

100. Pearson CA, Ajayi AO, Okunyade MA, editors. *Training for General Medical Practice in Nigeria*. Ibadan: University of Ibadan Press, 1980.

101. McWhinney IR. Family medicine as a science. *Journal of Family Practice* 1978; **7**(1): 53–8.

102. Stewart M, Brown JB, Weston WW et al. *Patient-Centered Medicine: Transforming the Clinical Method*. 2nd ed. Oxford: Radcliffe Medical Press, 2003.

103. Haggerty JL, Reid RJ, Freeman GK et al. Continuity of care: a multidisciplinary review. *BMJ* 2003; **327**(7425): 1219–21.

104. Fortin M, Stewart M, Poitras ME et al. A systematic review of prevalence studies on multimorbidity: toward a more uniform methodology. *Annals of Family Medicine* 2012; **10**(2): 142–51.

105. Fortin M, Bravo G, Hudon C et al. Prevalence of multimorbidity among adults seen in family practice. *Annals of Family Medicine* 2005; **3**(3): 223–8.

106. Macaulay AC, Commanda LE, Freeman WL et al.; North American Primary Care Research Group. Participatory research maximises community and lay involvement. *BMJ* 1999; **319**(7212): 774–8.

107. Legare F, Stacey D, Turcotte S et al. Interventions for improving the adoption of shared decision making by healthcare professionals. *Cochrane Database of Systematic Reviews* 2014; **9**: CD006732.

108. Glanville J, Kendrick T, McNally R et al. Research output on primary care in Australia, Canada, Germany, the Netherlands, the United Kingdom, and the United States: bibliometric analysis. *BMJ* 2011; **342**: d1028.

109. De Maeseneer JM, van Driel ML, Green LA et al. The need for research in primary care. *Lancet* 2003; **362**(9392): 1314–9.

110. Mant D, Del Mar C, Glasziou P et al. The state of primary-care research. *Lancet* 2004; **364**(9438): 1004–6.

111. Canadian Primary Health Care Research & Innovation Network [homepage]. Available at: http://www.cphcrin-rcrissp.ca/ (accessed 30 November 2015).

112. Dibarboure-Icasuriaga H, Haretche A. Aspects of decentralized medical care in CASMU: distribution of users and physicians [Spanish]. *Revista Médica del Uruguay* 1988; **4**: 139–47.

113. Grupo Médico Migues. La práctica médica general en un medio rural: aspectos epidemiológicos del asma 1977–1979 [General medical practice in a rural area: epidemiological features of asthma: 1977–1979] [Spanish]. *Revista Médica del Uruguay* 1985; **1**: 5–14.

114. Harzheim E, Starfield B, Rajmil L et al. Consistência interna e confiabilidade da versão em português do Instrumento de Avaliação da Atenção Primária (PCATool-Brasil) para serviços de saúde infantil [Internal consistency and reliability of Primary Care Assessment Tool (PCATool-Brasil) for child health services] [Portuguese]. *Cadernos de Saúde Pública* 2006; **22**(8): 1649–59.

115. Shi L, Starfield B, Xu J. Validating the Adult Primary Care Assessment Tool. *Journal of Family Practice* 2001; **50**(2): 161.

116. Grupo PCAT.UY; Pizzanelli M, Ponzo J, Buglioli M et al. Validación de Primary Care Assessment Tool (PCAT) en Uruguay [Validation of the Primary Care Assessment Tool (PCAT) in Uruguay] [Spanish]. *Revista Médica del Uruguay* 2001; **27**(3): 187–9.

117. PCAT.UY [homepage/blog] [Spanish]. Available at: http://pcatuy.blogspot.com/ (accessed 30 November 2015).

118. Centro de Investigación Epidemiológica y en Servicios de Salud. Colaboración IA-PCAT [Spanish]. Available at: http://ciess.webs.fcm.unc.edu.ar/grupo-ia-pcat-2 (accessed 30 November 2015).

119. Rubinstein AL, Irazola VE, Poggio R et al. Detection and follow-up of cardiovascular disease and risk factors in the Southern Cone of Latin America: the CESCAS I study. *BMJ Open* 2011; **1**(1): e000126.

120. Rodríguez Domínguez J, Fernández Ortega MA, Mazón JJ et al. La medicina familiar en México, 1954–2006. Antecedentes, situación actual y perspectivas [Family medicine in Mexico, 1954–2006. Background, current situation, and perspectives] [Spanish]. *Atención Primaria* 2006; **38**(9): 519–22.

121. Gómez Clavelina FJ. Formación de investigadores en Medicina Familiar: estrategias y retos [Spanish]. *Atención Familiar* 2006; **13**(3): 69–70.

122. Deo L. Primer foro de investigación en Medicina Familiar de la ALPMF [Spanish]. *Archivos en Medicina Familiar* 2007; **9**(1): 19–22.

123. González Pedraza Avilés A, Velasco Jiménez M. La importancia de la investigación en el primer nivel de atención a la salud [Spanish]. *Revista de Especialidades Médico-Quirúrgicas* 2008; **13**(4): 149–52.

124. Ramírez Aranda JM, Gómez Gómez C, Flores Fuentes EL. Productividad en investigación por médicos familiares y generales [Spanish]. *Revista Médica del Instituto Mexicano del Seguro Social* 2003; **41**(2): 175–80.

125. Fajardo-Gutiérrez A. La publicación y su compromiso con la sociedad [The publication and its commitment to the society] [Spanish and English]. *Revista Médica del Instituto Mexicano del Seguro Social* 2014; **52**(4): 364–66.

126. Diogene Fadini E. *Guía de investigación clínica para atención primaria.* Ediciones Mayo, Barcelona España, 2005. Chapter 1 Investigación en atención primaria: Situación. Parte I – Estado actual y perspectivas futuras de la investigación clínica en atención primaria; p. 3–16 [Spanish].

127. Suarez Cuba MA. La investigación en la atención primaria de salud [Spanish]. *Revista Médica La Paz* 2010; **16**(1): 3–4.

128. de Noronha JC, de Araújo Oliveira J, Donato Rodrigues R et al. Transformações de um ambulatório de medicina integral com vistas a um programa de atenção médica primária: a experiência do Hospital de Clínicas da Universidade do Estado do Rio de Janeiro, Brasil [Reorganization of an outpatient dispensary aiming at a Primary Health Care Programme: experience of the Rio de Janeiro University Teaching Hospital] [Portuguese]. *Revista de Saúde Pública* 1977; **11**(4): 429–43.

129. Rosenthal R, Jacobson L. *Pygmalion in the Classroom: Teacher Expectation and Pupils' Intellectual Development.* New York, NY: Holt, Rinehart & Winston, 1968.

130. Paim J, Travassos C, Almeida C et al. The Brazilian health system: history, advances, and challenges. *Lancet* 2011; **377**(9779): 1778–97.

131. Gusso G, Pérez Fernández M, Gérvas J. Brazilian health-service organisation: problems at a glance. *Lancet* 2011; **378**(9788): 316–17.

132. World Organization of National Colleges, Academies, and Academic Associations of General Practitioners/Family Physicians. *Classificação Internacional de Atenção Primária (CIAP 2)* [Portuguese]. 2nd ed. Florianópolis: Sociedade Brasileira de Medicina de Família e Comunidade, 2009. Available at: http://www.sbmfc.org.br/media/file/CIAP%202/CIAP%20 Brasil_atualizado.pdf (accessed 29 November 2015).

133. Macinko J, Guanais FC, de Fátima M et al. Evaluation of the impact of the Family Health Program on infant mortality in Brazil, 1990–2002. *Journal of Epidemiology & Community Health* 2006; **60**(1): 13–19.

Index

Entries in **bold** denote boxes and tales; entries in *italics* denote figures.